# Relaxation
## ON THE RUN
by Jay Winner, M.D.

Simple Methods to
Reduce Stress in Seconds
*plus*
Practical Lifestyle Tips
for a Happier and Healthier Life

## Acclaim for Jay Winner's books:

*"A great teaching, simply presented. It's practical, wise, and truly valuable for a healthy life."*
Jack Kornfield, Ph.D., author, A Path with Heart

*"Practical, useful, and effective."*
Dean Ornish, M.D., author, Stress, Diet, and Your Heart and Love and Survival

*"I highly recommend this book and CD set as a wonderful, easy way to decrease your stress and improve your health. It is an entertaining read packed with important and useful information."*
Jack Canfield, cocreator, the Chicken Soup for the Soul series

*"A practical guide to a happier and healthier life, that inspires us with hopeful examples."*
Richard Roberts, M.D., J.D.
past president, American Academy of Family Physicians, and past president, World Organization of Family Doctors

*"A terrific guide—accessible and immensely practical—for dealing with the largest everyday problem of modern times. Dr. Winner makes a stress-free life seem within our reach. Honestly, I learned a lot myself!"*
Diana Winston, director, Mindfulness Education, Mindful Awareness Research Center, UCLA, and author, Wide Awake and Fully Present

*"This is one of the most comprehensive books on stress reduction out there. Dr. Winner brings lightness to a heavy topic. He shows us how to deal with our human condition of stress and suffering with insight, wisdom, and a good dose of humor. He uses mindfulness to help people see options for a better life. There is something for everyone in this book."*
Elissa Epel, Ph.D., associate professor, UCSF, Dept. of Psychiatry

"Being a healthy person in today's world means knowing how to manage stress, and this resource is a must-have. Jay Winner has compiled a great book on everything you ever wanted to know about stress and how to live in joy!"

Cherie Carter-Scott, Ph.D., author,
*If Life Is a Game, These Are the Rules*

"Dr. Winner covers an amazing amount of material in a reasonably few number of pages. In doing so he takes on a fascinating variety of roles. He is part family doctor, part psychologist, part meditation teacher, part inspirational speaker, part cheerleader, and part friend. As if that were not enough, the way he writes is better than all of those combined. His sincerity, honesty, and humility are compelling, and his relaxed, conversational, anecdotal writing style renders this information accessible to everyone— including the type of person who would never read, much less enjoy, a book on stress management. This book is an easy read. I will give it to my patients because I trust they will enjoy it and therefore will be much more likely to follow its suggestions than those in most of the other stress management books I have read."

Larry Bascom, Ph.D., psychologist and past president,
Santa Barbara County Psychological Association

"Although there are now myriad resources about stress management, most either focus on one method or provide an overview that is either too esoteric or too simplistic. Dr. Winner has accomplished the significant task of integrating all of the major contributions to stress management in a very readable manner. His book provides thoughtful and pragmatic one-stop shopping for readers who wish to better manage stress and to improve the quality of their lives."

Steve Shearer, Ph.D., cofounder,
Anxiety and Stress Disorders Institute of Maryland

"A great user-friendly book. A must for any health resource center, hospital library, medical clinic, or patient education department."

Dawn O'Bar, coordinator, Sansum Health Resource Center

"I had the pleasure of seeing Dr. Winner present two outstanding workshops on stress management — one to General Dynamics and another to mental health professionals. I found his approach extremely valuable and relevant to my work as the director of an employee assistance program. One leaves his presentation armed with an array of pragmatic and helpful stress management tools, which I now often share with my clients. His book nicely complements his thorough presentations. Without hesitation, I highly recommend Dr. Winner's stress management book and lectures/workshops."

Tom McIlmoil, director, Employee Assistance Services,
Santa Barbara Cottage Hospital

"Perfect for sale in a pharmacy. Reading this book makes customers' wait times go quickly, so we keep copies of Stress Management Made Simple at the front counter. We get tremendous feedback from customers and have trouble keeping it in stock."

Steve Cooley, pharmacist and pharmacy owner

"Two accompanying audio CDs offering guided meditation, stretching advice, and relaxation techniques complement Stress Management Made Simple, an excellent antidote to the immense stresses of 21st-century life as offered by author, medical doctor, and stress management instructor Jay Winner, M.D. From learning how to manage anger and frustration, to improving the quality of one's sleep, to simply better enjoying one's day, Stress Management Made Simple is an easy-to-read, reader-friendly, highly recommended addition to self-help reading lists, self-improvement reference library collections."

Midwest Book Review

# About the Author

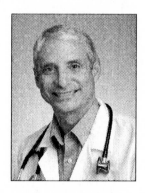

**Jay Winner, M.D.**, is a family physician and stress expert who has helped thousands of patients deal with stress. He is the founder and director of the Stress Management Program for Sansum Clinic, one of Central California's largest medical clinics. Dr. Winner has spoken on the topic of stress management to corporations, physician groups, counselors, military personnel, and government employees. He has written articles for professional medical and counseling journals, and is often quoted as a stress expert in a wide variety of national print and electronic media. He lives in Santa Barbara, California, and was the chairman of the Department of Family Medicine for Santa Barbara Cottage Hospital.

*More information about Dr. Winner and his work is available at www.stressremedy.com*

PUBLISHED: May 2015, edition 2015
Blue Fountain Press,
Santa Barbara, CA

Designed by Anna Lafferty,
Lafferty Design Plus, Santa Barbara, CA

ISBN:    978-0-9745119-1-7

NOTE:    The information in this book is true and complete to
the best of our knowledge. This book is intended only
as an informative guide for those wishing to know
more about health issues. In no way is this book
intended to replace, countermand, or conflict with
the advice given to you by your own physician.
The ultimate decision concerning care should be
made between you and your doctor. We strongly
recommend you follow his or her advice. Information in this book is general and is offered with no
guarantees on the part of the author or publisher.
The author and publisher disclaim all liability in
connection with the use of this book. The names and
identifying details of people associated with events
described in this book have been changed. Any
similarity to actual persons is coincidental.

*This book is dedicated
to my family, friends, patients,
students, and teachers.*

# CONTENTS

# INTRODUCTION

## *If I had the time for a stress management class, I wouldn't be so stressed!*

As a family doctor who runs the stress reduction classes for one of the largest medical clinics in Central California, I've heard that sentiment more than once – and it's very understandable. By now, many people are familiar with the harms of excessive stress, such as increased risk of heart attack and obesity. Perhaps they even know that too much stress can age them, shorten their lives and double their risk of Alzheimer's disease. They may realize that the overabundance of stress can sap the joy from life and worsen almost any medical problem. And they *think* that the only solution lies in hours of meditation, Tai Chi or yoga – hours that they just don't have. No wonder they're frustrated.

What they don't know:

## *Some of the best stress reduction techniques can be done in seconds.*

The antidote to stress is relaxation and our society on the whole has a relaxation deficit disorder. Where do we lack sufficient relaxation? For some, their jobs are too tense, and a joyful, relaxed, efficient way of working seems as foreign as an obscure Martian dialect. For others, home life isn't the oasis of peacefulness they would like. For the other 98 percent, it's both of the above. Most of us would benefit from more relaxation both at work and home.

This book has three types of exercises to help you relax:

**1. RELAX ON THE RUN** These relaxation exercises take as little as two seconds and, at most, a minute. They are simple, fast and can be seamlessly integrated throughout your day. The key to these techniques is that *they are fast and therefore can be done frequently.*

**2. PRACTICE** Longer relaxation exercises provide a deep level of relaxation. *More importantly, they can help you practice and become more proficient* in the Relax on the Run exercises. With that in mind, I skipped exercises in which you imagine relaxing on a beach – those types of exercises might help you to chill a bit, but do you really need extra practice in the skill of beach relaxing? In contrast, all the practice exercises in this book build the skills that let you relax in the midst of a hectic day.

**3. LIFESTYLE TIPS** Although this book emphasizes the quick ways to decrease stress, it also covers some strategies that involve a little extra planning. A few small strategic changes in our environment and lifestyle can sometimes make a dramatic difference.

These three types of stress reduction are like three legs of a stool. If you're not an acrobat and try standing on a one-legged stool, or even a two-legged stool, you'll soon have a painful rendezvous with the hard ground. However, the "three-legged" strategy of relaxation on the run, practice, and lifestyle exercises provides the stability for a relaxed life.

For quick reference, many of the relax on the run and practice exercises are written in boxes, as are many of the lifestyle tips.

Think of this book as a relaxation and stress reduction tool kit. Have you ever, for lack of a screwdriver, tried to use an old butter knife to do the job? No? OK, then it's just me. Anyway, the dull butter knife doesn't always work, and replacing it with a good Phillips head screwdriver can turn an unworkable problem into a simple fix. Having the right tools on hand for tackling stress can let you easily relieve what previously had felt like a heavy burden. Not all tools will work equally well for everyone. Depending on your personality and circumstances, you will find certain ideas and techniques that fit you best. If one chapter does not seem helpful to you, please keep reading. One patient told me that the chapters on mindfulness changed her life, and another found that the chapter on communication skills made all the difference.* If you are a nutritionist, you might not learn a lot from the "Less Stress Nutrition" chapter, but a chapter on cognitive psychology may be key.

The Relaxation on the Run techniques are simple and straightforward. You'll pick up many of them right away with minimal effort. If some others take a little practice, no worries. A beginning violin student can make finger nails on a blackboard sound good in comparison. Yet with practice, playing beautiful music can become as natural as breathing. Every technique in this book is a thousand times easier than playing the violin. Many are easier than playing the kazoo. So with just a little patience, you'll be relaxing on the run. (And if not, there's always the kazoo.)

---

*Throughout the book there are stories to illustrate the points. To protect privacy, all names and some other identifying characteristics in these anecdotes have been changed.

This book will give you the information necessary to master these techniques. If desired, you can also explore supplementary audio material at www.stressremedy. com. Throughout the book, I'll point out when there is optional audio material available on a particular subject.

If you are already familiar with some of the topics, be patient with the process. Even experts benefit from going back to the basics and perfecting them. Tiger Woods, when he was heralded as the best golfer in the world, took time off to review basic stroke mechanics and emerged an even better golfer for it. I've taught hundreds of stress reduction classes, yet every time I teach a class, I'm reminded of ways to handle my own stress more effectively. In the same way, if you are already familiar with some of the concepts presented in this book, *Relaxation on the Run* should serve as an important reminder of vital skills that we all forget from time to time.

The funny thing is that I didn't initially set out to write a book. I didn't even set out to become a stress reduction teacher. I began my career in family medicine, and, like a typical family doc, I saw people with a wide variety of ailments. Even in the first year of practice, it became increasingly clear that many of these conditions were exacerbated by stress. I could give my patients a pill for their headache or heart disease, but if I didn't address their stress, I was only treating a small part of the problem.

However, as a typical family doctor, I had perhaps fifteen minutes to address all of a patient's concerns, such as diabetes, chest pain, cough, and dizziness. How could I fit in talking about stress reduction? Except for brief discussions, I couldn't. What then?

"What then" happened in 1992 – with knowledge I had gained from multiple courses and books on psychology, counseling, stress management and meditation, I began teaching stress reduction classes. The first class was so well received that I scheduled another, then another. The written notes for the class helped class members and patients who were too busy to make it to class. Those notes were the "seed," which after more than 30 years of studying stress reduction, and 23 years of teaching people fast and efficient ways to relax, developed into this book.

Whether you have an average stress load or you're as anxious as a hummingbird on espresso, *Relaxation on the Run* will help reduce your stress. You would not expect to work at almost any profession without instruction. You would not expect to run a marathon without training your body. In order to live the most joyful life possible, it makes sense to get some basic instruction and training in relaxation. My students have ranged from people with minimal stress to people with full-blown anxiety disorders. Virtually all of them come away with useful stress-reducing skills.

Congratulate yourself for starting the journey to a healthier and happier life. If you make the commitment to finish the book and follow through with the recommendations, you will be able to relax on the run.

# 1
# Relaxing Quickly

The first skill in reducing stress has to do with breathing, which is not as controversial as you might think. In fact, 19 out of 20 doctors strongly recommend that their patients breathe on a regular basis. The other 1 out of 20 are medical examiners who do autopsies – they get kind of freaked out when their patients breathe.

When we're anxious, we often breathe shallowly, relying on muscles around our ribs and necks. As any opera singer will tell you, to get a deep, full breath you need to use your diaphragm – a big dome-shaped muscle that separates the chest from the abdomen. When the diaphragm contracts, this dome starts looking a bit more like a pancake – it flattens out. By doing so, the lungs can fully expand. At the same time, the diaphragm pushes down on the organs in your abdomen and those organs need to go somewhere. We have a spine and can't just get taller with each inhalation, so with each diaphragmatic breath the abdomen expands. (See Figure 1)

With each inhalation, gently let your abdomen expand. (If you have a little trouble with this, you can try diaphragmatic breathing while lying down, perhaps with a light object on your abdomen.) As long as your abdomen expands, it's fine if your chest expands as well. As you breathe slowly and gently in this fashion, you may start feeling more relaxed.

In order to improve the degree of relaxation, let go of your current thought and just feel your breath deep in your abdomen. Pay attention to your abdomen expanding with a full inhalation and then relaxing with a full exhalation.

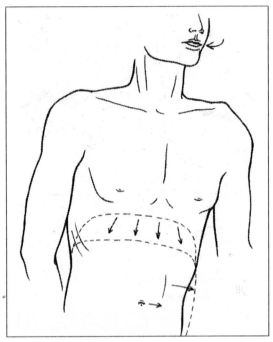

FIGURE 1: With each breath in, the diaphragm
contracts and flattens, forcing the abdomen out.

**Relax on the Run**

## DIAPHRAGMATIC BREATHING

Let any thoughts go and feel your abdomen expand
with a full inhalation. Then feel it relax and recede
with a full exhalation.

An advantage to this Relax on the Run exercise is that
the duration of one breath is brief enough that it enables
us to pay full attention. Focusing without distraction for
fifteen minutes – that's tough. Doing it for a breath or
two – you can do that! To make the relaxation even more
effective, it helps to pay attention to your body.

## Relaxing the Body

In Western culture, we tend to think of the mind and the body as separate entities. Well, let's test that theory. Think of a time when your body was extremely tense, but your mind was relaxed. Having a bit of trouble? How about a time when your mind was in turmoil and extremely anxious, but your body was hanging loose? Coming up a bit short? Of course you are. You've got a spinal cord that connects your brain to your body.

If you want a relaxed body, you can do it by relaxing your mind. If you want a relaxed mind, relax your body. And if you do one of the exercises in this chapter that relaxes both your mind and body at the same time? Now we're talkin'!

---

**Relax on the Run**

### MINDFUL INHALATION MUSCLE RELAXATION

This exercise is useful since it can be done quickly and in any posture: sitting, standing, or lying down. So, you've got zero excuses for not doing it right now. With each inhalation, feel your abdomen gently expand outward. With each exhalation, relax a different muscle group. For instance, with the first exhalation, you might relax your jaw and the muscles around your mouth; with the second, your neck; with the third, the little muscles between your eyes; with the fourth, your shoulders; and with the fifth exhalation, your back. If a thought comes into your mind, just let it float by and feel the next full inhalation in the abdomen and with the exhalation, let a new muscle group relax. It will not be long until you are feeling more calm and at ease.

*Seth's blood pressure was good at home but higher at work, and even higher at the doctor's office. After doing this exercise for about 30 seconds, his blood pressure dropped 23 points.*

If you are in real rush, just focus on one inhalation and relax your most tense muscle group with the exhalation. A lot of people have a "favorite" muscle group to tense – maybe your jaw, neck or shoulders. If you have a favorite, it will be well worth the four seconds it takes to focus on a mindful inhalation and then focus on relaxing that favorite muscle group on the exhalation.

*Sam was 17 years old when he came to see me. He was having recurrent headaches and nausea. He hated taking medications and wanted to explore other treatment options. Sam experienced stress about several different issues in his life, such as his high school basketball games. Typically, he would feel a little nervous, wish he felt differently, and start clenching his jaw. Soon his headache would begin. After we talked, Sam tried another approach. As soon as he felt himself starting to get stressed or wishing he felt differently, he would let the thoughts go, focus on diaphragmatic breathing, and relax his jaw. By the time of our next visit, Sam's headaches were occurring much less frequently.*

## Relaxed Posture

This book is all about easy. Rather than struggle with a complex ballet pose, relax with a simple valet pose. Figure 2 shows an old-time piece of furniture called a clothes valet. It looks like a horizontal clothes hanger sitting atop a vertical pole. The shoulders of shirt are supported and the rest of the shirt hangs as it would on a regular hanger.

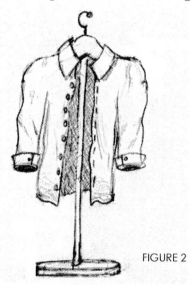

FIGURE 2

### Relax on the Run

### VALET POSE

Stand with your back straight and your shoulders back. Keep your head up. Imagine that your spine and shoulders form the clothes valet, all the rest of your body is like a shirt that hangs loosely off the valet. Got it? Spine straight, shoulders back, all the rest of your muscles soft and loose. Your face, jaw, forehead, arms, legs ... all soft and loose. Get a real sense of what your whole body feels like in this posture.

In two seconds, you can assume the valet pose. Feel your body with spine straight, shoulders back and your other muscles soft and loose. And if you like, throw in a little smile and/or diaphragmatic breath for good measure. This exercise is helpful since you relax your body while keeping a healthy posture. That way you can be relaxed without looking and feeling like a pot of mush.

Remember, the Relax on the Run exercises are fast, so they can and should be done frequently throughout the day.

---

**Relax on the Run**

## MOVEMENT

You don't have to turn into a statue to be relaxed. You can have that same sense of an upright spine and relaxed muscles as you walk, dance or stretch.

---

**Relax on the Run**

## WHOLE BODY/FULL BREATH

Just another variation on the theme. Feel your whole body in its entirety as you take the full inhalation and full exhalation.

---

## Squeegee Breath

For some, another visual image may help with relaxation. Dr. Dike Drummond, physician coach and health care speaker, recommends using the image of a squeegee – tool of window washers or people who are compulsive about clean shower doors.

## SQUEEGEE BREATH

As you inhale, "feel" the breath go to the top of your head, hold your breath for two seconds, and then as you exhale, imagine a squeegee going down from your head cleaning away all muscle tension and distracting thoughts.

## Touch

How else can we use our body to relax? Hmm ... Should I go there? Why not? Sensuality! Our sense of touch – and not just when you're doing the bedroom samba. There are many other experiences worthy of recognition. For most of human history, an indoor warm shower was unheard of. Imagine someone who has never had a warm shower feeling the jets of warm water on their skin for the first time. You probably shower every morning, but are you so busy obsessing about this or that, you don't feel a drop of water?

## SENSE OF TOUCH

Practice noticing your sense of touch and the variety of pleasant experiences it delivers. Enjoy a shower, feel your feet on the ground, the toothbrush massaging your gums, soap sliding as you wash your hands, the warm pressure of a hug, and the list goes on. At least for a moment, let go of your current thought and just feel. Even a couple of seconds devoted to noticing your sense of touch will relax you.

Remember, the Relax on the Run exercises are fast so they can be done frequently throughout the day. If you take just five seconds to do one of these exercises sixty times throughout a day, the total time spent that day would be five minutes. Every Relax on the Run exercise is like buying a share of Apple stock in 1980. Tiny investment of time and effort – relatively huge payout in stress reduction.

Some of these exercises may resonate more than others for you. Pick out a few of them, such as mindful diaphragmatic breathing, mindful inhalation muscle relaxation, valet pose, and focusing on the sense of touch – then sprinkle the exercises throughout your day.

Now that you've got a handful of relaxation on the run skills, it makes sense to learn more about stress. After all, before you can master something you need to understand the basics.

# 2

# Good & Bad Stress

*"Adopting the right attitude
can convert a negative stress
into a positive one."*

Hans Selye,
pioneering stress researcher

Imagine a prehistoric man sauntering across a grassy savannah. Out of the corner of his eye, he sees a massive saber-tooth tiger. Boom! Instantly, hormones are released in the man's body that make his heart pound faster, his breath quicken, his pupils dilate, and his blood rush from his gut to his muscles. For the next few moments, as his body is flooded with extra oxygen and energy, he is stronger, faster, and sharper than normal. Whether he fights or (smarter still) flees the ravenous tiger, this reaction may well make the crucial difference. If the man is walking with a friend who lacks this "stress response," the friend is more likely to become the special entree of the day. But our prehistoric man wins the 50-yard dash and survives to pass on his genes – and stress response – to future generations ... to us!

Yet why would this very reaction that saved our ancestor's life ruin ours? Stress enabled our forebearers to hunt better, live longer, and thrive. Why does it hinder our work, harm our relationships, and threaten our health?

Answer: the saber-tooth tigers have changed – they no longer have sharp fangs, bone-crushing jaws and devastating claws. Our saber-tooth tigers now appear as traffic jams, busy weekends - and overloaded work schedules. The stressful circumstances have dramatically changed, but the stress response is one in the same, having evolved as a physical solution to a physical threat. However, threats of our world are rarely physical, and a physical response is rarely appropriate. If work is hectic and you respond by punching your boss in the nose, you'll certainly get a pink slip, and maybe earn free accommodations – at the local jail.

An overnight stay in jail would not be the worst problem from stress. We should be so lucky! During a four-year study, people with high levels of stress had a 63 percent greater risk of dying than people with lesser stress. Stressed out and think a little wrinkle cream will reverse aging? Think again: In another study, women with a lot of stress had actual changes in their DNA – changes the equivalent of aging an additional 9 to 17 years. There is even research showing that people under high levels of stress have twice the risk of developing Alzheimer's disease.

You'd be hard pressed to find a medical problem not made worse by excessive stress, a small sample of which includes heart disease, obesity, headaches, acne, eczema, psoriasis, irritable bowel syndrome, and heartburn. Stress may also affect the treatment of diabetes, high blood pressure, chronic pain, and asthma.

On other fronts, a million folks in the U.S. miss work every day from stress-related disability – and millions more are much less proficient at their jobs because of stress.

Maybe you should blow off work and just stay in school? Also not a perfect plan; studies show that stress is the number one impediment to academic success.

So if I asked if you wanted stress, your response would likely be, "Are you crazy?" Most people think stress is as useless as an air conditioner in an igloo. The burst of adrenaline helped the caveman avoid being lunch, but surely today life is different. Nowadays, we need stress like we need dinosaur-hunting gear, right?

The truth is that the stress response is as much a part of us as is our heart or liver. When the system is working well, it can help us accomplish important tasks. One night I was sound asleep when I was awakened by the sound of my then-five-year-old son screaming. I did not get out of bed in the usual fashion. From a sound sleep, I vaulted over my wife and made it down a flight of stairs and to my son's side in less than five seconds. When I got there, I discovered that the emergency was that his covers had fallen off. I then explained to my progeny that "covers falling off" is not a reason to call the National Guard, dial 911 or, more importantly, interrupt my sleep. However, the point is that I could not normally have accomplished that vault, stair descent, and run in five seconds. With the help of an adrenaline burst, I was able to do it from a sound sleep. And if there had been a real emergency, those precious seconds could have made all the difference.

If you are tired and are either taking an exam or playing a sport, a little extra adrenaline can actually improve your performance. But indeed, there can be too much of a good thing. Too much adrenaline earns an "F" on your exam and isn't so great for your tennis game, either.

In short, a certain amount of stress can be helpful. We call this good stress *eustress*. The extra energy or adrenaline is often felt as excitement, passion, and enthusiasm. When we exceed our stress quota, however, we enter the land of *distress*. That's often felt as anxiety, and a tight knot in your stomach. Other signs of distress are muscular tension, fatigue, racing heart, insomnia, irritability, shakiness, excessive sweating, upset stomach, lack of appetite, and a sense of being overwhelmed.

Stress is most useful when there is a short burst of energy that can help us accomplish a task. Excessive and prolonged distress can lead to myriad health, relationship, and work performance problems. And, of course, it feels miserable. With high levels of prolonged stress, not only is too much adrenaline released, but excessive amounts of the hormone cortisol are also spewed from your adrenal glands. Cortisol can decrease inflammation, but it also has some less desirable effects. It decreases your immunity and makes it harder to fight off infections. It makes you ravenous (supposedly to make up for the calories you burned in "fight or flight") and encourages storage of the new calories as belly fat – the very type of fat that is associated with diabetes, heart disease, and stroke. To complicate matters further, if adrenaline has your motor running way over the recommended RPMs for a long time, you're on the expressway to the junk heap. It's time for an overhaul, before it's too late.

Throughout this book are various strategies for relaxing and reducing stress. Let's look more in depth at what really puts the "dis" in distress, and how you can convert distress into good stress, or eustress.

Many people like roller coasters, but not all enjoy the beginning of the ride. Your palms get sweaty, your heart pounds, and your pupils dilate. You quietly (or not so quietly) cuss the friend who talked you into taking this stupid ride. When you reach the top of the roller coaster and look down that first big hill, you're convinced you're going to die. However, as the ride continues, you find yourself excited and enjoying the swift turns. Wait a minute – what happened? The adrenaline is still flowing through your bloodstream, your heart is still pounding fast, your palms are still sweaty, and your pupils are still dilated, but now you're having fun. What's different?

At the beginning of the ride, maybe you wished that you were somewhere else and that your body wasn't so tense. But by the middle and end, you just accepted the ride for what it was and enjoyed the rush. In other words, as you stopped resisting the experience, your anxiety was transformed into excitement.

Now say the word *eustress* slowly out loud. *Eustress* sounds a lot like *use stress*, doesn't it? And that's a good way to think of it. How many performers have gotten up in front of thousands of people and never had a surge of adrenaline? Probably not many. The good ones learn to use that excess energy. At times, it is best to handle stress by using the additional energy to be excited and to enthusiastically pursue your goals.

Although not all stress is bad, the statement "I'm stressed" has a very negative connotation to most people. Just the thought of being stressed can lead us to resist our feelings. In turn, the more we resist stress, the more distressed we get. In a sense, we get anxious about being anxious. Solution? One strategy is to replace the thoughts

"I'm stressed" or "I'm stressed out" with the thoughts "I have a high energy level" or "My adrenaline level is up" and then to use the energy. Remember, the original purpose of the stress response was to not only alert us but also to give us a robust physical boost. Even if you don't actively "use" the energy, you can, in a sense, welcome it.

---

**Relax on the Run**

## USE STRESS

1. When you feel stressed and you are in an appropriate setting, see how it feels to say to yourself, "Great! I have a high energy level." Let go of any thoughts to the contrary. Assume the attitude of being thankful for the extra energy. Then turn on some music and dance, or go out for a run with some upbeat music on your MP3 player. You will likely find this activity works to convert the distress to eustress.

2. The next time you feel stressed, try again saying to yourself, "Great! I have a high energy level." Feel the desired energy course through your veins. This time, proceed doing your normal activity with this extra energy.

There are many ways to relax. Sometimes you might enhance that relaxation by listening to mellow music. At other times, you might use the stress and sing and dance to an upbeat tune. Either way, by not resisting stress, relief is possible.

---

A 2012 research study brought further clarity to the topic of converting distress into eustress. In that study, three groups were monitored as they performed stressful tasks, including public speaking and doing math in front of disapproving evaluators. Even if the participant spoke as eloquently as Martin Luther King, Jr. and did math problems like a savant, he was treated to a barrage of frowns, furrowed brows and disapproving negative feedback. Prior to the tasks, one group had an easy unrelated task, and another was advised that the best way to deal with the stress was to ignore the external cues (frowns, negative feedback, etc.). The final group was given some reading that suggested that the stress response evolved over the years as a useful adaptation – instead of being harmful, the readings suggested stress would help one accomplish tasks. In the authors' words, the last group was told to "reappraise arousal."

In all three groups, the heart output increased – no surprise there. Here is the interesting thing: In the first two groups, when under stress, the blood vessels constricted, making blood flow more difficult, while in the reappraisal group the blood vessels dilated.

How can we make any evolutionary sense of this difference? Perhaps the first two groups mimicked an animal (or early human) in a hopeless situation – they might not outrun danger and needed to limit bleeding, while people in the reappraisal group mimicked ancient hunters needing a boost in performance to overcome their prey.

For us though, the reason for the difference is less important than the implications of the difference. I would not go out of my way to seek out stressful circumstance just for the sake of being stressed. However, if you are in a stressful circumstance, resisting and wishing away the stress just compounds it and makes it more harmful – resistance turns the stress into distress. Accepting the stress as potentially helpful and using the energy can turn it into eustress.

In other words, often the best strategy is to *choose to use stress*. Properly channeling your stress makes you happier and healthier, and it can improve your performance in physical and mental tasks. The following chapters on mindfulness will make this even clearer, and they will give you tools to create a richer and more relaxing life.

# 3

# Mindfulness

*"In order to be utterly happy, the only thing necessary is to refrain from comparing this moment with other moments in the past, which I often did not fully enjoy because I was comparing them with other moments of the future."*

Andrê Gide,
author and Nobel laureate

Enjoyable, healthy activities, such as hiking, bathing, eating, watching a sunset, and listening to music, are good for you and can help you relax. However, if you obsess about your problems as you participate in these activities, the benefit will be minimal. Eating a healthy gourmet meal can be relaxing and pleasant. However, if you're too preoccupied, the food will be bloating your stomach before you've ever really enjoyed a bite. Playing tennis can be a relaxing activity, but if you're so angry about a missed shot that you want to send your racket into orbit – not so relaxing.

Which brings us to the questions of the day:

1. How can you make your relaxing activities truly relaxing?

2. How can you make your stressful activities less stressful and more enjoyable?

The answer, in one word or less is *mindfulness*.

## The Present Moment

Simply put, mindfulness involves non-judgmentally focusing your attention on the present moment. To begin exploring the concept of mindfulness, consider this question: "How many ways can this present moment be?" You don't need a degree in astrophysics to answer this question. Over time you can affect a change in the environment. You could move from point A to point B. You could build new relationships, maybe get another job, buy a bowtie, whatever. But this very moment can only be the way it is. Nevertheless, the average person spends a tremendous amount of time wishing that the present moment were different. As soon as the alarm goes off in the morning, a stream of thoughts begins: "I wish I didn't have to go to work today." Unless you don't have a job and then think, "I wish I could go to work." "If only it weren't so rainy out." Unless your area hasn't had rain for a while and then: "If only it would rain." "I wish the kids would be quieter." And if you don't have children, "It would be great to hear some children happily playing." When it's not "I'm too busy," it's "I'm too bored!" Are you getting the picture? Our ability to relax is hampered by our uncanny ability to complain to ourselves.

Why are we stressed in a traffic jam? All we have to do is follow the driver in front of us. A trained monkey could do that. The stress is a lot less about the traffic and a lot more about our thoughts. Most likely, we are saying or thinking something to the effect of "I wish I weren't stuck here ... What bad luck I have ... I can't be late ... " And there may be a few words like: "#&**!" and "*%*#!" to boot. You're convinced that the driver ahead of you is either evil incarnate or a drunken baboon. We'd have to change the very fabric of the universe for the present to be any different than it is. But that doesn't stop us from emphatically wishing for it.

Let's compare that miserable traffic jam with life at its best. Think of a peak experience, those wonderful times when life seems perfect or even spiritual. Perhaps holding your newborn for the first time comes to mind. Maybe you're thinking of a time when you were looking over the scenic Yosemite Valley. I wonder what would have happened if you took the previous traffic jam mentality and overlaid it upon your peak experience:

- First time with your newborn: "What an ugly baby! My cousin got a much cuter one."

- Yosemite: "Half dome? Couldn't we afford to go to a place with full dome?"

What made your peak experiences the wonderful events they were was that you were not dwelling on thoughts like the ones above. All peak experiences have a common element: They occur when you are fully present, enjoying the moment just as it is, as opposed to wishing that this or that were different.

Back to the traffic jam: When you have the thought "This traffic jam is horrible," you don't have to believe it. You don't have to give yourself a hard time about it. Instead of getting lost in your ruminations, let the thought go and enjoy a breath, and/or feel your body (remember the "valet pose") or listen to relaxing music on the radio. Couldn't be simpler: Let the thought go and enjoy a present moment sensation. And it's awesome that this technique is so easy – you can repeat it 30 times in a 15-minute period ... without even breaking a sweat.

## FOCUS ON THE PRESENT

If you have a thought about the present being different, let the thought go and focus on a present moment sensation like breath, body, sound or taste. You don't have to believe a given thought. Some of your thoughts may be fact, but many are just opinions and judgments.

I was asked, "How do you let thoughts go?" Some analogies might be helpful here: You don't have to do any work to let a cloud float overhead and you don't have to labor to let a leaf flow down a stream. Similarly, it takes no effort at all to let a thought go. Thoughts come and go on their own all day long. By paying attention to the present moment, extraneous thoughts just disappear. In essence, what may sound like a two-step process of letting go of a thought and then focusing on the present is really a one-step process. Just focus on the present.

If your mind drifts to thoughts of how this moment needs to be different, all that is necessary is to pay attention. Non-judgmentally attend to the current breath, to body sensations, to sound, to taste or even to your thoughts. Don't worry if a particular negative thought occurs frequently. The skill lies in seeing how quickly you can focus back on the present moment just as it is. Be patient. Be gentle to yourself. Be kind. Each time your attention wanders, it gives you an additional opportunity to practice an extremely important skill – refocusing on the present. If a thought comes up 100 times, that's fine – you've got 100 times to practice.

## A Few Thoughts About Thoughts

I wrote about letting thoughts go, but let's get one thing straight – I do not intend to bad-mouth thinking. Before humans acquired thought, we were up a creek without a paddle. Then one of us thought, "How about using a paddle?" Without the ability to think, we'd be trying to get around with square wheels and building with round bricks. Thought is what helped us emerge out of the Stone Age and into the computer age (with a step or two in between).

Even our daydreams are not so bad. Some researchers feel that much of our creativity comes from our non-purposeful thinking. When we need that creative solution, our daydreams may help connect the dots between two apparently disparate items to come up with a unique, out-of-the-box answer. (In fact, when a creative solution eludes you, focused concentration on the computer screen might not bring an answer. Changing your scenery with a walk outside may stimulate new thoughts and new solutions.)

So thinking is important – but non-stop? Really? An essential ingredient for a relaxed joyful life is spending some time fully and mindfully enjoying the present moment. When we are lost in our thoughts, the thoughts determine our reality. When we think, "I'm having a bad day," the day is indeed bad. The process of noticing our thoughts as thoughts is called decentering. When we take this figurative step back, it opens up the possibility of not having to believe all our thoughts. We can let certain thoughts go, refute certain thoughts, dance with thoughts, whatever. We can also find joy in the space between our thoughts. And, we can think more purposefully towards solving our goals.

## Goals

Practicing mindfulness certainly doesn't mean abandoning all goals. Without goals, we would accomplish very little. There are times when it is appropriate to think about the future and to make plans. When we are mindful, we learn from our past and plan our future, but, by not obsessing on either, we do not lose sight of the present moment.

We can and should work to make changes in the future, but in doing so, we should also challenge ourselves to enjoy the process. Theologian Reinhold Niebuhr wrote, in the often-quoted serenity prayer, "God, grant me the serenity to accept the things I cannot change, Courage to change the things I can, and the wisdom to know the difference." I would add, "Please give us the understanding that change often takes time, and the wisdom to enjoy the process of change." In other words, we should use mindfulness as a tool to enjoy the journey.

Without mindfulness, life can become a never-ending series of desires, with little enjoyment of the here and now. While in high school, we can't wait to graduate and enter college. As college students, we want to graduate. When working, we might wish for retirement. When we're old and retired, we'll likely yearn for the "carefree" days of childhood. Maybe we think that life will be better if we are married; or if we're married, we think that divorce will bring us happiness. If happiness were achieved only when our goals are met, our happiness would be short-lived indeed, since another "goal" is always around the corner.

> **"For a long time it had seemed to me that life was about to begin—real life. But there was always some obstacle in the way, something to be got through first, some unfinished business, time still to be served, a debt to be paid. Then life would begin. At last it dawned on me that these obstacles were my life."**
>
> Alfred d'Souza, clergy

The ability to make and work on goals is an essential tool for a productive life. Thinking that happiness is achieved only by meeting all your goals is a recipe for a miserable life.

## Mindfulness and Stress

Even a small increase of mindfulness can dramatically improve the way that you handle stress in your life. Figure 3 illustrates an escalating stress problem. The first small stressor may be no big deal. However, just like walking up the Empire State Building is done one step at a time, stressor after stressor can bring the adrenaline level to a dizzying height. When this high level of stress is sustained for long periods, physical and emotional prolems are likely to arise. In contrast, each time you bring yourself to enjoy the present moment, even for a short period of time, you decrease your  level of stress (see Figure 4). Every moment you are  mindful not only brings more relaxation to that moment, but also decreases the stress in the moments that follow. As Figure 4 demonstrates, with relatively few added moments of mindfulness, the stress fails to reach the high level in Figure 3. It is unrealistic to expect that you will be mindful 100 percent of the time. However, an increase in mindfulness from one percent to just two percent of the time doubles your stress reduction.

Figure 3

## Level of Stress

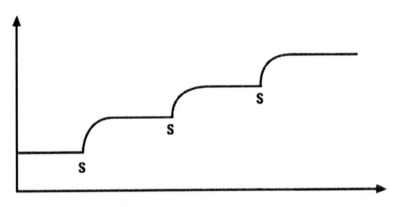

S = Stressful incident
Stress is more harmful when it continues to rise
and stays elevated.

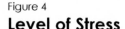

## Level of Stress

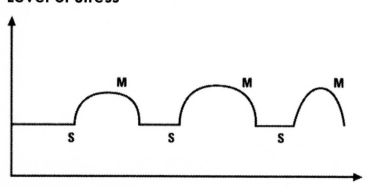

S = Stressful incident
M = Moment of Mindfulness
As you can see, even a few episodes of mindfulness
make a significant difference in how you handle stress.

## The Stress Cycle

When something bothers you, it seems natural to resist or try to push it away. A rock rolls into your path, and you push it back to where it came from. With stress, that strategy doesn't work well. Often people elevate their anxiety level by trying to resist their anxious feelings. They get anxious about being anxious – stressed about being stressed.

Imagine pushing outward at a door that is pushing against you. The more you push, the more the door seems to push back and no matter how hard you push, you can't open the door. That's how we often fight stress – hard work and you just feel worse. What I'm suggesting is to stop pushing at the door. Just stand aside and the door will open inward and you can walk through. Figure 5 illustrates how we often resist stress and shows how the cycle is as unproductive as pushing on a door that says "Pull."

Figure 5

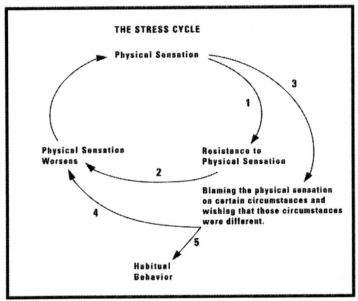

A common physical symptom of stress is feeling your heart pounding fast, so I'll use that sensation as an example. If you don't like the feeling, it's natural to resist the sensation and wish your heart would slow down (Figure 5, Arrow 1). "I hate how I feel. I hope my heart slows down! It's going way too fast." Guess what happens next? That's right – your heart goes faster. Resist more – your heart races even faster; resist more and before you know it, your heart is speeding at Warp 5. (Figure 5, Arrow 2). In addition to this cycle, another cycle may ratchet up the stress. For instance, you might blame your anxiety on your supervisor's actions. If you focus your thoughts on wishing that your boss behaved differently, you end up resisting the present circumstance (Figure 5, Arrow 3). Your heart rate and anxiety then further increase (Figure 5, Arrow 4).

Some people attempt to relieve stress with a habit, such as smoking, nail-biting, or overeating (Figure 4, Arrow 5). These habits do not arise out of a thoughtful decision; it's usually not, "Hmm. What would improve my situation? Yes, that's it. If only I had thought of it before. If I chew my fingernails down to the cuticles, that will solve the problem." The habit more likely comes about when your mind is busy complaining about a topic unrelated to the behavior, and then lo and behold, you look down and where there had been fingernails there are now only remnants. Or where there had been a full bag of Doritos now stands an empty foil of cheese dust. Instead of paying full attention to what you are doing, most of your focus is on your thoughts. So while most of your mind is otherwise preoccupied, your body is left to fend for itself. And thereby, you rely on a habit that may yield a limited degree of temporary relief – even if it exacerbates the problem in the long run.

Some people may try to solve the problem by being critical of their thoughts, but that can be another losing proposition. As you berate yourself for unconsciously decimating an entire large pizza, you create more suffering – so now you're upset and giving yourself a lecture – a perfect setup for even more automatic behavior providing short-term relief in exchange for long-term turmoil. If you lecture yourself about too many thoughts, those thoughts multiply and quickly spin out of control..

There's got to be a better way. When a patient comes to me complaining of a racing heart, I start by asking enough questions to reassure both of us that the sensation is not caused by a medical problem.* If the racing

---

* See Chapter 24 for more information.

heart is caused by anxiety, as it frequently is, I tell my patient to focus on his breath and let his heart beat as fast as it can. This is not because I want to hear "Flight of the Bumble Bee" through my stethoscope. By letting his heart beat as fast as it likes, while taking some mindful diaphragmatic breaths, the heart actually slows down. Resistance is what fueled the vicious circle described in Figure 5. No resistance means no vicious circle.

Similarly, making a conscious effort not to resist external circumstances, such as your supervisor's behavior, can also decrease your stress level. Maybe you can change your boss's future behavior with some tactful feedback. However, for the present moment, focusing on the wish that your boss would currently be different delivers more fuel to that same heart-race cycle.

If you notice yourself engaging in an automatic behavior or habit, it's a signal that you are probably not being mindful. Pay attention to the physical sensations and the thoughts that tend to occur with, or before, that behavior. Let the associated thoughts go as you focus on your breath. Rather than "running away" from the uncomfortable physical sensations by grabbing a cigarette, gorging on junk food, or turning on the television, try to sit with the feeling for a few moments. By accepting the knot in your stomach and taking some mindful diaphragmatic breaths, you may find that the discomfort decreases or passes altogether. Taking that little break may be enough to let you make a wiser choice, and not bite your fingernails down to the knuckles, or smoke those death sticks, or stuff unneeded calories into an already full stomach.

## BREAKING THE STRESS CYCLE

Ideally, break the stress cycle as soon as it starts. Don't spend 20 minutes wishing things were different. As soon as you notice a "resistant thought," bring your attention to your next breath (or other present-moment sensation). If the thought comes up again, patiently let it go. Remember that the more thoughts you have, the more practice you gain in mindfully refocusing your attention. Be patient with yourself. Each time you realize that your mind has drifted, be thankful for that realization and bring your attention back to the present. By learning to recognize the thoughts and feelings of stress early, you can break the stress cycle before it starts, or at least before it goes very far.

*"In Spring, hundreds of flowers,*
*In Autumn, a harvest moon,*
*In Summer, a refreshing breeze,*
*In Winter, snow will accompany you.*
*If useless things do not hang in your mind,*
*Any season is a good season for you."*

Mumon Ekai, Zen master

Notice that the poem did not say, "If useless things do not come to your mind." It said "hang in your mind." How we deal with the thoughts that we have can bring us back to enjoying the present moment.

Put another way:

> **"***That the birds fly overhead,***
> ***this you cannot stop.***
> ***That they build a nest in your hair,***
> ***this you can prevent.***"**
>
> Ancient Chinese Proverb

Thoughts will certainly fly around in your mind. The trick is to notice your thoughts as just thoughts. You don't have to believe your thoughts and there is certainly no reason to resist your thoughts. Doing so may provide too much "nesting material." On the other hand, if you're patient with yourself, you can easily refocus on this moment – full of beautiful flowers, harvest moons, and refreshing breezes.

In the next chapter, we'll discuss specific effective methods to relax deeply when you have a few spare minutes. We'll also discuss how these same exercises will prepare you when you don't have those spare minutes.

# 4

# Practice Makes
# ~~Perfect~~ Better

A common way doctors test the heart is a stress treadmill test. You walk and then run on a treadmill with a bunch of wires connected to your chest. Picture this: About a decade ago, I'm getting a treadmill test (I won't keep you in suspense; it came out fine). I'm working hard, panting like a dog and sweating like, well, like an animal that sweats a lot.

The cardiologist tells me I can stop. He's satisfied that my heart rate was high enough for the test. But I wanted the test to be as accurate as possible, so I really wanted to get my heart rate to the max. Perhaps my misplaced competitive nature also pushed me to want to run on. So I say, "Why don't I keep going a little longer? If I have a heart attack from exertion it's best to have it right in front of a cardiologist." The cardiologist replies, "I'm not worried about you having a heart attack. I'm worried you might trip and break your leg."

For most people, watching someone have a heart attack would be going straight to Panicville. For a cardiologist, dealing with a heart attack is relatively routine. The difference is that the cardiologist has had a lot of practice with dealing with heart attacks. He is prepared. However, his last experience treating a broken bone may have been decades ago in medical school.

Another example of preparation is the virtuoso musician. An expert cello player has much more of his brain dedicated to the control of his left hand. All those hours of practice actually add many more nerve cells and nerve cell connections dedicated to the control of the hand. If you had told this to a neurobiologist in 1985, he would have laughed at you for being so mistaken. Tell that to a neurobiologist today, and he will laugh at you for bothering to state such an obvious fact. The reason for this is the acceptance of a concept called neuroplasticity. The dogma in 1985 was that by the time you're born, you have most of your adult brain cells and certainly by the time you reach adulthood, the brain cells and connections are all set; as unchangeable as the past. As it turns out, scientific doctrine changes and so do our brains. Neuroplasticity means that our behavior, environment and even our thoughts can change the function and even the structure of the brain.

With practice, the musician builds the brain connections to make playing his instrument second nature. In the same way, with some practice, you can become a virtuoso in relaxation. Dealing effectively with anxious feelings will be as easy as Yo-Yo Ma playing "Mary Had a Little Lamb" on his cello.

Throughout the day, each time you are mindful, bringing your attention fully to the present moment without judgment, it strengthens those connections in your mind. The more you practice mindfulness of breath and body sensations through the day, the more natural it is to be mindful.

As far as "practice makes perfect" – well, that's what we call a "high bar." Although we will never be mindful anywhere near 100 percent of the time, practice will strengthen your skill of quickly refocusing on the present moment.

Being mindful during the day is vital. Extra practice is also very helpful. Imagine difficult times in life as a juggling a chainsaw, machete and lit torch – all while riding a unicycle. In your life the chainsaw might be a work emergency, the machete – paying the bills, and the torch – problems with your family life. Think of meditation as tennis balls. Juggling tennis balls and you drop them? Just pick them up again. Drop the chainsaw on your leg (or make a big mistake at work) – it's more complicated than that. Just as it makes sense to practice juggling with tennis balls to improve your skill, it makes sense to practice being mindful when mindfulness is your only task. Then you'll be more prepared for challenging times.

Perhaps another analogy makes more sense to you. Meditation is like:

- **practicing** your groundstrokes so they are second nature at your big tennis match.

- **practicing** your piano scales so that you can later master that difficult piece.

- **practicing** your times tables so that the more complicated math problems are easier.

In all these cases, we get good at the basics in a low-demand environment, and then are ready to meet the challenge in higher-demand settings.

## BREATH AND BODY MEDITATION

When you can spare anywhere from five to twenty minutes, take some time to get some more intense practice. Sit up with nice posture and focus on one breath, then another, and another untill your mind drifts to your work, or perhaps your homelife, or to thinking "Why am I wasting my valuable time noticing my breath?" Sooner or later a thought will pop up – that's fine; it's all part of the exercise. When you realize that you've stopped paying attention to your breath, you have a few different choices:

1. Go back to another group of thoughts. Maybe "Oh yeah, I was supposed to be meditating. On the other hand, there is some really blah blah blahbabbity in the yada yada..."

2. Give yourself a hard time: "What a loser I am. I got distracted only after one breath. This is almost as bad as the time when I thought a ZIP code was a secret signal that my fly was open."

3. Blame the technique, thinking, "This doesn't work. So what if millions and millions of people have been meditating for several thousands of years? They should have talked with me before wasting their time!"

4. Be grateful that you noticed that your attention drifted and gently bring it back to your breath.

At one time or another, you'll probably do all four of these options, but the point is to practice #4 – be grateful that you noticed your attention drifted and gently bring it back to your breath. You really can't bring your focus back to the breath until you, in a sense, "wake up" and notice that your attention has drifted. So be grateful for that moment, and patiently bring your focus back to the sensation of this one breath.

Below are a few more hints for times of body/breath meditation:

1. View your meditation sessions as a reward – as time you set aside for yourself. Be grateful for the time to deeply relax. Even if a particular meditation session seems frustrating, the practice will still deepen your ability to relax during the day.

2. Don't struggle or try hard to relax. Struggling to relax is a bit of an oxymoron, don't you think? Just follow the instructions in this chapter and your practice will be beneficial. In fact, it's not a bad idea to have a bit of a smile as you meditate. The smile reminds you not to be too serious.

3. When you're first learning to meditate, find a quiet setting. With more experience, you may benefit from the challenge of a noisier setting. You can let any noise be a signal for you to go deeper into your meditation.

4. You may need to be creative in finding times to meditate. Like exercise, you can use meditation as you need it. However, there is much benefit to incorporating meditation into your daily routine. Perhaps, when the alarm goes off in the morning, instead of hitting the snooze button several times, sit straight up in bed, and do a meditation to start your day. Alternatively, right after work or before dinner may be a good time for you.

5. Get comfortable. You can sit in a chair with your legs uncrossed and your hands flat on your lap, sit on a

pillow on the floor, or lie on your back. One disadvantage – or perhaps, advantage – of meditating lying down is that you may fall asleep during the meditation. Falling asleep may be an advantage if it is time to go to bed, but a disadvantage on a workday morning. If you are sitting as you meditate, assume a comfortable yet upright
posture – keep your back straight and shoulders back.

6. Start with mindful diaphragmatic breathing. I find it most useful to focus on the sensation of the breath in the abdomen. Other options could be feeling the breath in the nostrils, throat or lungs. You might even feel your whole body in the process of breathing. Pay attention to the full duration of the in breath and the full duration of the out breath. Don't analyze or think about the breath. The idea is to focus on and enjoy the sensation of just this breath. To convey this, people have used descriptions such as "tasting the breath" or even "luxuriating in the breath." If you find that diaphragmatic breathing is too difficult or uncomfortable, then just watch your breath as it is. As you become more relaxed, you may find you are naturally breathing using your diaphragm.

7. As mentioned before, when thoughts come to mind, do not resist them. Instead of judging the thoughts, just notice them, and then gently let them go. Perhaps imagine each thought as a cloud floating by, or a branch floating down a stream. If you have an abundance of thoughts, do not be discouraged. Meditation is not about having zero thoughts, but about developing your ability to gently refocus your attention. When you've noticed that your mind has

drifted, patiently bring your attention back to your very next breath – feeling the entire inhalation and the entire exhalation. Don't be surprised if your meditation sessions initially consist of a lot of thinking and only a few minutes focused on the breath. A transcript of your thoughts during a meditation might read: "I have a bunch of chores to do. I also need to get a lot of work done tomorrow – oh yeah, I'm meditating... I wonder what time ... My back ..." Don't worry; as long as you learn to gently let the thoughts go and focus on your next breath, the meditation is working.

8. Avoid resisting your body sensations. Sometimes the more you resist an uncomfortable sensation, the more spasm you create in the surrounding area. When you stop resisting the sensation, sometimes the discomfort eases.

9. After you've been practicing mindful breathing for a bit, you may want to begin paying attention to your body. Relax one part of your body at a time, starting either with your feet or with your head and working your way along your entire body. You may then refocus your attention to your breath. Then get a sense of mindfully feeling your whole body in the process of breathing.

10. Another potential tool for meditation is the use of a repetitive phrase, sometimes called a "mantra." In general, people like to choose soothing sounds like "om" or "one." Others like meaningful words such as "love" or phrases like "be here now." Some people will use one word or phrase with the inhalation and

another with the exhalation. Zen master Thich Nhat Hanh mentions using "Breathing in I calm myself; breathing out I smile," or the shorter "calm; smile." Lately, my favorite mantra has been "one," since "one" is actually a twofer. It is soothing and very meaningful. An abstract meaning some people might give "one" is that when your mind is quiet, illusions of separateness fall away and all people, and in fact all the world, seems as one. But it's way too early in the book to get that deep, so try this: When you meditate, all you need to do is pay attention in this one moment to this one breath. Saying this very short word reminds you to just enjoy this one full inhalation and one exhalation. Some people with a religious tradition may like to repeat a short prayer as a mantra. There may be another phrase that you find comforting. Have you ever heard a song in the morning and had it run through your mind throughout the day? In the same way, a meaningful mantra may become a useful reminder of mindfulness throughout the day.

11. Generally, it is best to continue the meditation session uninterrupted. If you occasionally have very important thoughts, you can keep a notepad and pencil nearby. If you decide to do this, however, you should rarely use the notepad. The notepad becomes useful if otherwise you would be spending 20 minutes worried about forgetting, or actually forgetting, an important responsibility (such as picking someone up at the airport).

12. I recommend starting your meditation practice with your eyes closed. Later, if you prefer, you can try meditating with your eyes open. When your eyes are

open, you can maintain an unfocused gaze or focus on an object, such as a flower, a candle, some artwork or just a scenic view.

13. If you'd like, you may end the meditation with a phrase, such as giving thanks for the present moment, the people in your life, your health, and so on.

14. How long to meditate? That largely depends on your schedule. Some experts recommend meditating 20 minutes twice a day or 40 minutes daily. If you can regularly find that time, excellent. However, I'm in the camp that it is better to find five to ten minutes to meditate once or twice a day than try for a 40-minute meditation, but only do it once a week.

15. When you are first learning to meditate, it is helpful to do a guided meditation. If you meditate without a recording, consider using a timer so you know when the meditation is over. That way you do not have to keep checking your watch. Any timer will do, but there are a variety of timers explicitly for meditation. These timers tend to have a pleasant bell or chime to signify the end of the period. (Using a loud buzzer is probably not a good idea for obvious reasons.) There are CDs used to time meditation, smartphone apps, stand-alone timers, and free online meditation timers.

16. Like most skills, meditation improves with practice and dedication. Just as it takes time to build your muscles with physical exercise, your ability to focus will improve as you exercise it with meditation. Do not expect one meditation session to be like another. It is helpful to continue your regular practice despite

any thoughts of boredom or discontent. There is a great deal to be learned from meditating when your mind is distracted. Learning to deal with distracting thoughts in meditation will teach important skills that can be used throughout the day. Buddhist nun and author Pema Chödrön said, "I've had many times when I meditate, and it seems like my mind is just going 100 miles an hour. And yet, when I stand up and walk into life, there's more room in my mind."

When does meditation fit into your day?

**Optional Audio Exercises** of six-minute and twenty-minute guided meditation available at www.stressremedy.com

# 5
# Putting Mindfulness into Practice

## Using the Right Yardstick

How about using your car odometer to measure the width of a dime? You don't need to be a mechanical engineer to understand the futility of that task. It is important to use the right tool and units of measurement for a particular task. Want to measure evolutionary changes? You can probably forgo the stopwatch. If you want to measure the time to complete a college degree, a good unit of measurement is years. Want to measure the length of a movie, hours would be the way to go. So what is the appropriate unit of measurement for mindfulness? This one moment. This one breath. This one footstep. This one bite of food.

Bummed out because you're having trouble being mindful for 20 minutes? Quit using a yardstick to measure the size of an electron. If you think that mindfulness is hard, it's because you are using the wrong unit of measurement.

Alcoholic Anonymous has helped many with its 12-step programs. One of its helpful core principles is "one day at a time." This principle is helpful in strengthening one's ability to keep away from alcohol or to keep on a diet. However, for the purposes of mindfulness, "one day at a time" is 23 hours, 59 minutes, and 58 seconds too long. The principle for mindfulness is "one moment at a time."

> ### Relax on the Run
> ## THE ONE-BREATH CHALLENGE
>
> Let's do an experiment. On the count of 3, pay attention to one inhalation and one exhalation – that's right, just one breath. Ready, 1 . . . 2 . . . 3: go.
>
> Were you able to do it? If not, try again. OK. You've now demonstrated that you can be mindful without any problem. The next time you have a thought that it is difficult, you can let that thought go and fully focus on the next breath.

## Beginners

Our society does not glamorize the beginner. If you're planning to have brain surgery, are you going to deliberately choose the surgeon who is a beginner? Probably not. If you bet on a sports match, is your money going on the professional or the beginner? Unless the pro just had both of his knees broken, you know the answer to this one. So the beginner loses out again ... but not always.

Two people are watching a play. One is an usher at the theater, and therefore has seen the play 200 times. The other is a novice who has never seen the play before. Which of them is likely going to enjoy the play more? The award here would likely go to the beginner. The beginner has more curiosity and interest. The usher is likely listening more to his own thoughts than to any dialogue on stage.

It's easy to see how the toddler would really enjoy his first experience walking on a grassy lawn. He looks at the grass, smells the grass, and feels the grass. Us, on the other hand? We likely don't even see the yard. We're thinking about work, or perhaps wondering what's for dinner. We don't experience the yard. When you experience something for this first time, sometimes mindfulness seems more natural.

But when you've seen thousands of lawns, how can you enjoy it as much as the first-timer? Let go of your thoughts and come back to your senses. Feel the grass under your feet. See the rich green color, enjoy the fragrance. And thus, you bring the advantage of the beginner's mind to the experience. A really great basketball player has learned to bring full mindfulness and focus to each shot. In that way, he combines the skill of an expert with the attention, focus, and curiosity of a beginner.

Think back to your mindful breathing meditation. Meet each breath with a curiosity and interest – treat each breath as a unique entity. And when you get good at enjoying your breath, staying interested in almost any other setting should be a piece of cake.

Experience something as if it's new. If you're on your front lawn, take off your shoes and feel the soft grass on your feet. Look at a flower and notice each petal. Brush your teeth like it's the first time – feeling the bristles massage your gums, tasting the toothpaste, and even hearing the sound of the brush.

---

**Relax on the Run**

## BEGINNER'S MIND

What are you doing right now? Do one small step at a time with the joy and novelty of a beginner. If right now the task is scrubbing the floor, watch how the water changes the floor's color with every stroke. Whatever you are doing, meet this moment with curiosity.

## Have Some Sense

*"The purpose of life is to live it, to taste experience to the utmost, to reach out eagerly and without fear for richer and newer experience."*

Eleanor Roosevelt

When it's late at night and I just want my dog to hurry up and pee, I'm thinking, "Quit sniffing around and just pee already. It's not rocket science." However, I could more easily understand rocket science than discern the different smells that form my dog's world. For all I know, when my pup smells a patch of grass, she may be checking out the equivalent of doggy-Facebook – keeping up with the news of the neighborhood dogs. Certainly, my dog's keen sense of smell would make her experience of the world much different from mine. Indeed, our experience of reality is largely formed through our senses of sight, sound, touch, taste, and smell.

Our senses can also have another function – they can be relatively easy access points to mindfulness. So far we've mainly discussed the sense of your body – the feeling of your body breathing, awareness of parts of your body, awareness of your whole body, and sensation of touch. Other doors to mindfulness include sound, smell, sight, and taste. It's as simple as letting go of thoughts of how life should be and hearing this one sound, smelling this one fragrance, seeing this one sight, or tasting this one bite of food. We'll cover the senses of taste and smell in more depth later.

## MINDFULNESS OF SOUND AND/OR SIGHT

As your mind wanders, you may bring your awareness back to the sounds of running water, or birds, or music. If you let go of your judgments, you can find music in the mundane. The hum of an engine or children playing can also potentially be music. Have you listened to a song one day and found it boring or even annoying, yet another day found it enjoyable? Evidently, at least part of our enjoyment lies in not only what we listen to but also in how we listen.

Similarly, look at a beautiful picture or gaze at a flower or an outdoor scene. As judgments come to your mind, let them go and enjoy the scenery. As you develop this skill, scenes you may have previously ignored suddenly seem worthy of a painting.

**Practice**

## SOUND AND/OR SIGHT MEDITATION

Start with the meditation on breath (as described earlier). After several minutes, try expanding your awareness to the sense of your body. And then, after several more minutes, pay attention to meditation to sound. Let go of any judgments of the sound and just listen. When you notice that your mind has drifted away, practice gently bringing the attention back to sound.

Similarly, you can meditate with your eyes open and bring your focus to some scene. Perhaps you might focus on a candle, a rose, or some outdoor scenery. When your attention wanders, patiently bring it back.

## Thought and Beliefs

As mentioned earlier, our perception of reality is filtered through our senses. If you were a dog, your sense of smell would take a more dominant role in your view of reality. If we had echolocation, such as a bat or dolphin, our sense of reality would also be altered – and you wouldn't bang your knee on that low table in the middle of the night.

However, our senses are not the only filters of reality. Our thoughts and beliefs also filter our perception. If you believe that your co-worker is rude, you'll look at all his actions through that filter. If you're sure that country music is bad, as soon as you perceive music as country, you will likely be prejudiced against it.

As we discussed earlier, the process of decentering involves noticing your thoughts as thoughts and your emotions as emotions. Instead of believing all your thoughts, you have the freedom to notice them. Instead of "There is no way to deal with my boss," you realize it's just a thought and that there are other ways you could perceive the world. In this way, you are not the victim of your unexamined beliefs and thoughts.

---

**Practice**

### WATCH THOUGHTS

Close your eyes, focus on a few breaths. Then focus on your thoughts. Instead of getting lost in your thoughts, watch them go by like events. When you try watching your thoughts, you may notice that no thoughts arise. That is interesting in its own right.

---

---

**Practice**

## MINDFULNESS MEDITATION

In this exercise, start with the breath meditation described earlier. Then, after a few minutes, expand your awareness to your body. Then notice sounds. Then notice thoughts and emotions. Finally, non-judgmentally notice anything that comes into your awareness – be it breath, body, sound, thought, smell, or emotion. This type of practice is the one that most closely mimics mindful awareness during day-to-day life. As another option, you can start with awareness of sound and expand your awareness to breath, body, thought, emotion, and, finally, to everything.

---

**Relax on the Run**

## MINDFULNESS OF DAILY LIFE

Take the sense of being fully present that you learned and practiced in the last exercise and bring it to your daily life.

---

**Optional Audio Exercise:** mindfulness of sound, breath, body, thoughts and emotion available at www.stressremedy.com

## Naming

Naming your thoughts, emotions, and physical sensations, as they arise, is a tool that can foster mindfulness. For instance, you can say words to yourself such as sadness, thought, or neck tightness, as one of those events happens. If you like, you can be more specific, such as noting "financial thought." At times, this process may help you focus your attention more easily and observe how your thoughts, emotions, and physical sensations come and go.

Most importantly, this naming or noting of a thought or emotion is not complaining. The noting is done in a welcoming fashion. The stress from obsessive thoughts is not so much from the thoughts themselves, but is more from resisting the thoughts. By welcoming all comers, the thoughts no longer carry such force. If some of the thoughts occur frequently, welcome them as an old friend. Another way of saying this type of noting would be "greeting." When welcomed (or noted or greeted) in this way, you realize that thoughts are very transient; they come and go like waves in the ocean. In the same way, when we note/greet an emotion, we are less likely to get stuck in that emotion, and, instead, we are more likely to flow from one emotion to the next. In fact, just the act of naming an emotion in this way seems to modify the reaction in a primitive part of the brain called the amygdala.

---

**Relax on the Run**

## NAMING AND GREETING

When you're meditating or feeling distress in the midst of the day, try just naming (in a welcoming way) your thoughts, emotions, and body sensations.

---

### *The Guest House*

*This being human is a guest house.*

*Every morning a new arrival.*

*A joy, a depression, a meanness,*

*some momentary awareness comes*

*as an unexpected visitor.*

*Welcome and entertain them all!*

*Even if they're a crowd of sorrows,*

*who violently sweep your house*

*empty of its furniture,*

*still, treat each guest honorably.*

*He may be clearing you out*

*for some new delight.*

*The dark thought, the shame, the malice,*

*meet them at the door laughing,*

*and invite them in.*

*Be grateful for whoever comes,*

*because each has been sent*

*as a guide from beyond.*

Rumi

## Reminders

You have an important event and you want to be sure to remember to go to it. What do you do? Of course, you give yourself a reminder. Whether in a written calendar, smart phone, watch alarm or string around your finger, when something is essential to remember, a wise person creates reminders.

Which leads to the next question: "Isn't being mindful and fully enjoying your life important enough for some reminders?"

There are two broad categories of reminders:

1. Specific reminders added to your day. This could include a sign on your desk reminding you to be present or an alert on your phone or computer. Perhaps you might wear a bracelet that reminds you to be more present.

2. Common everyday events. Examples of this might be taking a mindful breath every time you see a red light while driving. When your phone rings, you might take a mindful breath before answering the call. What activities do you do regularly that could be a reminder for you? As a physician, mindfully feeling my breath as I listen to a patient's lungs is quite natural. (More so than, say, sitting cross-legged and chanting "om" in the middle of a visit.) Since health care professionals wash their hands after seeing each patient, that can be a signal to feel the warm water and soap. If someone's job involved frequent trips to the copier, the act of copying might be a reminder to be mindful.

**LIFESTYLE TIPS**

## REMINDERS OF MINDFULNESS

What reminders of mindfulness would work for you? Ideas for signs, artwork, computer or smartphone reminders:

1. _____

2. _____

3. _____

4. _____

What activities do you do or what events do you participate in that could be reminders to be mindful:

1. _____

2. _____

3. _____

4. _____

Another way to make a reminder more effective is with practice. We talked about meditation as practice, and a variety of activities can be made into meditations. One friend told of her years as a Buddhist nun. One of the practices they would do was opening doors mindfully; time and time again, she would practice opening a door, while mindfully feeling the arm movements. Now, each time she opens a door, she is reminded to be mindful.

## Practice

### MAKE ROUTINE ACTIVITIES INTO MEDITATIONS

Is doing the dishes a normal part of your day? Instead of dreading the chore, wash one dish at a time. Enjoy the sensation of your hands in the warm, sudsy water. When you iron a shirt, bring your mind back from wherever, and watch the changes in the appearance of the fabric that occurs with each stroke of the iron. You can make these and many other routine activities into meditations.

For most of us, a frequent routine activity is walking. Why don't you use this time as a chance to practice mindfulness?

## Practice

### WALKING MEDITATION

There are several ways to perform walking meditation. One way is to bring your focus to your lower body – feeling the lifting and placing of each foot as you walk. As your attention wanders, bring it back to the sensation of your legs. You may feel the ground "massaging" your feet with each footstep. As opposed to thinking about getting somewhere, the idea is to enjoy the journey. Some of my students like saying the mantra "arrived" with every few steps to remind themselves that with each step, we have arrived at this moment. Another option is to practice mindfulness meditation as you walk, bringing non-judgmental awareness to your breath, your body, sounds, and sights. Most frequently, people start by walking slowly and deliberately. Later, you may apply this technique as you walk more quickly or even run.

**Optional Audio Exercise:** walking meditation available at www.stressremedy.com.

# 6

# When Mindfulness Seems Difficult

## When Justification Becomes Rumination

The first temptation when you are anxious and stressed is to resist the stress and wish it away. We've reviewed how well that works – not very. We've also reviewed how wishing the circumstances of life were different can increase the distress. Let's say you really want to make things worse. What can you do next? Since many people haven't learned to accept feeling anxious or sad, there is a natural tendency to justify the emotions: "Hmm ... I'm feeling anxious. Why is that?" And then you go on to list 30 reasons that could possibly explain the anxiety. "Work has been difficult. The children aren't behaving." And before you know it, reason number 30 reaches back to issues from your childhood. Now you can feel very justified in your anxiety. Do you see a problem here? Yes, listing all the things you could possibly be anxious about can only increase your anxiety.

"OK, OK," you're saying, "if I don't think about why I'm anxious, how can I correct it?" Good point. We do need to look at how we might improve our circumstances. However, it is very easy to go from solution-based thinking to counterproductive rumination. We need another alternative. And that, of course, brings us to mindfulness – learning to fully accept our emotions and physical sensations as they are.

*Samantha was participating in one of my stress reduction classes. She was having trouble with depression. I asked how she felt right now. She said she felt sad and wished she felt differently. Since sadness was not an acceptable emotion for her, she always needed to find justifications for being sad. These included recent problems and problems stemming from how she had been mistreated as a child. I asked if it was OK for her to let herself be sad. She said, "No. I hate being sad." I suggested that just for this moment, instead of resisting and justifying, she fully choose to feel whatever she felt. Then, 30 seconds later, I asked how she felt. She said, "Sad." Then, another 30 seconds later, I asked how she felt, and she no longer said, "Sad"; now she was relaxed. Usually her feelings of depression would last for hours. Samantha learned that trying to justify her feelings led to rumination and more depression. Instead, she could learn to be mindful.*

## Make Emotions Simple

**"It's like someone took a knife, baby, edgy and dull and cut a six-inch valley through the middle of my soul."**

Bruce Springsteen
singing "I'm on Fire"

Imagery makes poetry, literature, and music wonderful. If instead of the above lyric, Bruce Springsteen sang, "I'm sad," it wouldn't sell very many CDs. Metaphors, similes and complex stories of emotion help writers weave compelling and entertaining tales. It's no wonder we are tempted to tell our own stories in such elaborate terms. However, telling yourself the story of your own troubles with the dramatic flourish of a Shakespearean tragedy risks condemning you to suffering "the slings and arrows of outrageous fortune."

Consider someone going through a tough time thinking, "I feel horribly empty," or "I feel like I'm at the bottom of an endless pit." Seems a bit hard to be mindful of horrible emptiness or, even worse, being mindful at the bottom of a very deep pit. How can we not resist or judge such feelings? Let's begin by accurately and nonjudgmentally describing the experience. During the time we think "I feel horribly empty," we may see the emotion is sadness, and there is likely some physical sensation, such as a tight feeling in the abdomen. In addition to the thought "I feel horribly empty," there may be a series of other thoughts, such as "I can't take this any longer," and "I hope I feel better soon." When we mindfully register the sadness, it is fully experienced – and in the next moment, we are open to the next emotion. Perhaps it will be another shade of sadness; perhaps anger; perhaps joy. We are not stuck with being sad about being sad. We can then mindfully accept the physical sensation. (Even painful physical sensations are not as bothersome when they are mindfully attended to. This is why mindfulness training has been very useful for patients in chronic pain.) The thoughts can be noted as thoughts. When you don't believe or resist your thoughts, they come and go of their own accord.

As we pay keen attention to our emotions, we can observe that what we sometimes call an emotion is rather a thought, or a combination of emotion and thought. For instance, when we are meditating, we might say, "I feel like getting up now." It is probably more accurate to say, "I felt a tightness in my abdomen and had the thought that I wanted to get up." Then we can be mindful of the abdominal tightness and notice the thought as a thought. Similarly, when we are frustrated we might say, "I feel like escaping." This reaction might be described as, "I feel anger or frustration and I had the thought 'I feel like escaping.'" Another example is, "I feel overwhelmed." Likely, this could more accurately be described as, "I feel anxious and have the thought that I am overwhelmed." Still another example is, "I feel like having a cigarette." In that case, we could describe the thought of "I feel like having a cigarette" and investigate the true associated physical sensations and emotions.

When you are stuck, a useful exercise is to chart (on paper or just in your mind) the basic components of your experience. Break the experience into emotion, physical sensations, and thoughts. You might try using just the five emotions of happiness, sadness, anger, peacefulness, and high energy ("high energy" encompassing both anxiety and excitement, as explained in the second chapter). Even what is considered a common emotion such as loneliness can be examined more closely. Loneliness can be thought of as sadness with an implied series of thoughts about wanting to be with another person. If you wanted to use the five categories of emotion listed above, you might list frustration as anger with an implication that you wish something were different.

When you start talking or thinking about more complicated emotions, see if you can more accurately describe the thoughts, emotions, and physical sensations that are involved. When you say, "I'm empty," what does your body feel like? Perhaps there is heaviness around your eyes. Is the emotion sadness? What thoughts are there? Paying this type of close attention can help you become more mindful and not just lost in your thoughts.

**Practice**

## MINDFULNESS CHART

The chart starts with two examples. When you feel stuck, see if you can fill in the chart with some other examples. Feel free to make your own chart if you run out of room.

| Situation | Physical Sensations | Emotions | Thoughts |
|---|---|---|---|
| Have not heard from my friend | Tightness in neck | Sadness | I feel lonely. I wish my friend were here. |
| Work is very busy | Abdomen is tense. | High energy | Work is too busy. I wish I didn't work here. |
| | | | |

Accurately describing our emotions, physical sensations, and thoughts enhances our ability to be mindful. In summary, for songs, edgy, dull knives in the middle of your soul can be great. However, when you're mulling over your own life: Simple is better.

**Practice**

## THREE-MINUTE BREATHING SPACE

1. During the first minute, just assess what is going on currently: In simple terms, list your current physical sensations, emotions, and thoughts. Do not try to change them; just mindfully note them.

2. During the second minute, turn your full attention to your breath. Again, focus on the full duration of the inhalation and the full duration of the exhalation. Note where the breath seems easy to follow, perhaps at the nostrils or in the abdomen as it expands.

3. For the third minute, expand your awareness to include your body. Be aware of your whole body in the process of breathing.

   Keep in mind that you can use the ideas behind this technique for a shorter or longer "breathing space." Whether it's 10 seconds or 30 minutes, it can be beneficial.

**Relax on the Run**

## QUICK BREATHING SPACE

When three minutes seems like a long time (I know we've all been there), quickly go through the steps above in a minute or less

## Overwhelmed?

What do you do when you are overwhelmed? There is always the hyperventilate-in-a-corner-with-your-thumb-in-your-mouth option. I'm going to suggest a slightly different strategy.

Most of us have had the thought "I'm overwhelmed" at one time or another. Mindfulness teaches us to let that thought go and do what's next. For example, my first year of residency was one of my most stressful times. I might get called to see three people at once: Mr. A with shortness of breath, Mrs. B with chest pain, and Mr. C with leg pain. Rather than getting increasingly stressed, I let go of the thought "I'm overwhelmed" and focused my attention on taking care of one person at a time. I might ask Dr. Y to see Mr. A; then I would see Mrs. B, and then Mr. C. Alternatively, I might quickly check one patient to see that he was stable, then go to examine the next patient, and then return to the first. The point is to do what is next and focus on one thing at a time. The first task may be to come up with an attack plan, asking for help, or it might be starting right up with physical labor.

---

**Relax on the Run**

## DO WHAT'S NEXT

When you have the thought "I'm overwhelmed," let the thought go and do what's next.

*Richard was feeling progressively more anxious and overwhelmed at work. He said that at times, he felt like a "deer frozen in a car's headlights – too anxious to move." After we talked, Richard made a realistic plan of what he could accomplish at work and prioritized the tasks. In addition, he planned to notice the thoughts that occurred when he felt stressed. He might notice the thought "I'm overwhelmed." As soon as he noticed that thought, he would let it go and focus on his breathing, taking slow, diaphragmatic breaths. If the thought "I'm overwhelmed" came up again, he would again, patiently, let it go. As time went on, Richard also noticed thoughts such as "I don't like being here," "This is too hard," and "I hate this knot in my stomach." Each time he noticed one of these thoughts, he would let the thought go and focus on his breath. He would not resist the way his body felt. Instead of dwelling on everything he had to do, he would focus on doing the very next task. The more he did this, the more he found that he started enjoying his work and his stress decreased.*

## Not My Job?

The housing for a retreat was in dorm-style rooms, and the retreat was ending. I was supposed to finish cleaning my room before noon, but I got sidetracked. By the time I moseyed on back to do it, someone else had already finished the work. I meekly apologized, "I'm really sorry for giving you this extra work." However, the hard working stranger kindly responded, "There is no extra work; just work."

The task was not a problem for him. Another person

might have been very annoyed, thinking about the injustice of this extra burden and begrudgingly suffering through the "extra work." This fellow just did the work mindfully, focusing on the task at hand.

Are there two artificial categories you make: work and extra work? Perhaps we focus on doing one part of a job with ease and even enjoying it. Then there is the extra work, and the thoughts come: "Somebody else should do this. It is not my responsibility. I hate the paperwork. I should not have to work this late." By obsessing with these thoughts, we create much distress. What if, instead, we told ourselves, "There is no extra work; just work." We can let the thoughts go and focus on just enjoying the task at hand. That is not to say we should not try to change things. For instance, we might want to speak with a supervisor to change the required work, or we might want to delegate some of our work or figure out a way to decrease the paperwork. However, when we are right in the middle of required work, it helps to let go of the concept of "extra work" and just focus on the movement of our hand as we write, or the feeling of lifting the shovel as we dig.

## Mindfulness is Always Accessible

As you gain experience in meditation, you will soon appreciate its benefits. As things get stressful, you may think, "I need to meditate," or "I need to clear my mind." If you are tense, meditation will likely help. However, the above thoughts suggest that your feelings are not OK as they are. They suggest that you need to change to be all right. I strongly recommend that people regularly meditate. However, before meditating out of a need,

# "NOT MY JOB" LIST

Write down if there are tasks in your life that you make more difficult by thinking (in one form or another), "This is not my job" – that is, tasks that you tell yourself you would rather not do.

1. _____

2. _____

3. _____

4. _____

5. _____

Now, for each of those answers, take some time to reflect on two items:

1. Would it be best to delegate this task, or is there another way that you should relieve yourself of this particular duty? If so, make plans to proceed along those lines.

2. It may be best that you continue with the task. Or it may take some time to relieve yourself of the duty. If either of these statements applies, each time you have the thought "This is not my job" or "I don't want to do this," let the thought go and do the task with your full attention and care. Just enjoy each small step. What are the small steps that make up the task? If you are ironing shirts, iron each sleeve with care. If you are washing dishes, wash one dish at a time. If you are dictating a report, dictate with care, one word at time.

try just letting go of those thoughts and giving your full and complete attention to the full duration of an inhalation and the full duration of an exhalation (or another present-moment sensation). Being mindful takes only a moment and often gives you the perspective you need to deal with the stressful situation. You will find that if you then meditate with no immediate need or purpose, the meditation will be more fruitful.

## Learning to Let Go

The Letting Go meditation that follows serves several purposes:

1. This exercise experientially demonstrates that it is not just the thoughts but the belief in the thoughts that cause the emotional response.

2. This meditation gives people the practice in mindfully letting go of thoughts without needing to believe or resist the thoughts. Once that skill is learned, it can be applied in day-to-day life.

3. If a particular thought (either verbal or an image) has been emotionally charged, practicing this exercise can decrease the stress and fear associated with the thought. This exercise is particularly useful when learning to deal with obsessive and/or bothersome thoughts.

Learning to mindfully let go of certain thoughts is an important step in learning to manage stress and to thrive in life.

---

## LETTING GO MEDITATION

1. Start by following the meditation instructions in the prior chapter, namely mindful diaphragmatic breathing, letting go of thoughts and relaxing one muscle group at a time.

2. Certain thoughts (including ones that may have bothered you in the past) are then intentionally repeated. After repeating a thought (by saying the phrase to oneself), let it go and focus back on a mindful breath and relax a muscle group. The added instruction is to not believe or resist the thought, just let it go.

3. After going through this process, people usually become more relaxed. This demonstrates that stress results not from thoughts themselves, but from how we handle our thoughts.

---

**Optional Audio Exercise:** letting go meditation is available at www.stressremedy.com

*Michele suffered from panic attacks. These attacks were so severe and disabling that she often used medication for them. Just the thought of having an anxiety attack could trigger one. As she was watching a ball game, a friend joked that a new soda had so much caffeine it might give him a pan-*

ic attack. Michele then thought, "Oh, no! What if I get a panic attack now? I don't have my medication with me! That would be horrible!" And indeed, she became more and more anxious.

Michele came into the office for a brief appointment to discuss the panic attacks. I had her begin by focusing on diaphragmatic breaths. We did a meditation on breath. She started with letting go of her own thoughts. Then, I had her repeat the "charged thoughts" to herself (such as, "Oh, no! What if I get a panic attack now?"). Instead of fighting the thoughts or believing the thoughts, she was to notice them without judgment. She watched how the thoughts would come and go. She was instructed to just notice any sensations with interest and not resist the sensations. When the exercise was concluded, she was surprised that despite thinking her most scary thoughts, she was actually very relaxed. She learned that those "scary thoughts" did not harm her at all. She did not have to push the thoughts away. The thoughts were, in fact, flimsy and harmless. It was how she had "charged" the thoughts that had created the problem. She had charged the thoughts by believing them, and trying to resist them. Developing the skill of mindfully noticing her thoughts helped her effectively deal with her panic attacks.

For as long as Justin could remember, he had a problem with anxiety. One day, while under extreme stress, his heart rate jumped to 180 beats per minute and he was diagnosed with a heart rhythm problem called PSVT, or paroxysmal supraventricular *tachycardia. After that episode, his anxiety was far worse. Although he never had another episode of PSVT, whenever his heart rhythm was the least bit irregular he would start to panic. As he panicked, the rhythm would become even more irregular and uneven. Justin would start thinking, "I'm going to die. I hate how I feel. I wish this would stop." and so on. Justin needed to know how to deal with his thoughts and physical sensations. We did the Letting Go meditation He repeated the thoughts that troubled him, but, instead of resisting or believing the thoughts, he practiced just mindfully noticing them. He then focused on a diaphragmatic breath. Now, in addition to the medicine his cardiologist recommended, he had a tool to deal with his stress and did much better.*

## Always a Choice

On "Saturday Night Live," Roseanne Roseannadanna was puzzled: "Why don't people like saxophones and violins? What's all the fuss?" "No," she was told. The problem was not with "sax and violins," but rather "sex and violence." "Oh, never mind," she'd say, and then go onto her catch phrase, "It's always something."

And indeed, there is always something. At any moment, if we choose to, we can be creative enough to find something to be stressed about. If we choose not to be mindful, there is indeed "always something." If we try hard enough, we can always worry that we messed up in the past, or wish that the present were different. Even if things are going perfectly well, we can worry that our good fortune won't continue. At any given moment, we have the choice of whether to dwell on these thoughts or enjoy the present.

Our thoughts of discontent may seem to be unique, but they are usually nothing really special. They are likely to be very similar to thoughts we have had in our past and will have in our future. Within each moment is a test of how you want to spend that moment and, as the moments add up, how you want to spend your life. And through neuroplasticity, we know that each time we chose to be mindful, it makes that choice seem more natural in the future.

---

**Relax on the Run**

## CHOOSING MINDFULNESS

When you find yourself obsessing over a problem, ask yourself if this one issue is worth a life of distress. Wouldn't you rather have one of enjoyment? Set the precedent for how to handle the thoughts and issues in your life now. The only time you can choose to be mindful is right now. Do not waste this moment; choose mindfulness.

---

In the three chapters on mindfulness we covered a lot of ground, so perhaps it is time for the:

## Mindfulness Summary

1. The present moment can be only as it is, yet we spend a crazy-big amount of time wishing it were different. Predictably, this leads to dissatisfaction and distress.

2. Mindfulness involves deliberately paying attention to the present moment in a non-judgmental fashion.

3. The key to mindfulness is to patiently refocus your attention time and time again, then again and again, and then again ... Did I mention the being patient part?

4. As you make goals to change the future, realize that change may take time and let go of thoughts wishing that the present moment were different.

5. Resisting our physical sensations, thoughts and emotions just gets us stressed about being stressed. (Trying to reduce stress by resisting it is like treating your headache by banging your head against a wall.) To break that cycle, focus on a present moment sensation, such as the sensation of your current diaphragmatic breath. Perhaps tune into your body and relax a muscle group or two.

6. Each time you are mindful, it strengthens your tendency to be mindful. Whether it is in the midst of a busy day or during daily meditation, mindfulness practice is helpful.

7. Don't expect to be mindful for hours at a time. The right "yardstick" to use is mindfulness of this moment, this breath, this footstep, this bite of food.

8. Adopting a "beginner's mind" and tuning into your senses can help you be more mindful.

9. You don't have to (and shouldn't) believe all your thoughts. Because, face it – some of your thoughts are nuttier than peanut brittle. In the same way,

don't resist your thoughts – they come and go on their own accord, drifting away like clouds.

10. Sometimes just naming a thought or sensation in a friendly fashion will help you be mindful of it.

11. Set up reminders to be mindful. Some reminders may be in your natural environment, like your cell phone ringing, and others may be a sign or piece of artwork that you put up for the express purpose of being a mindfulness reminder.

12. Avoid justifying your emotions – listing the reasons for your anxiety, sadness or anger will just make those emotions more entrenched.

13. When you really feel stuck, consider simplifying your emotions and listing the basic emotion, thoughts and feelings. Doing a Three Minute Breathing Space can be helpful with this.

14. Overwhelmed? Let that thought go and do what's next.

15. Think one of your tasks is not your job? Either delegate it or accept it.

16. When you are bothered by repetitive thoughts or images, consider trying the Letting Go meditation.

17. Finally, remember that mindfulness is always a choice.

# 7

# The Lucky Sperm

Close your left eye and make your right hand into a tube. Now look through that tube at your left index finger. Bring the left index finger in close to the end of the tube so that the finger takes up most of your field of vision.

If you had a small wart on your finger, it would seem bigger now.

Now imagine that you were looking at the finger and wart under 100-fold magnification so that a tiny wart takes up almost your whole field of vision. Now the wart looks enormous – like it could swallow New York City – with grooves so large, you could build a new subway line in one. And a single ugly hair looks taller than the Empire State Building. Eeew!

Now, while keeping the ugly, humongous, NYC-eating wart in mind, let's talk about how our consciousness works. Our brains cannot focus on too much information at once. If we are in a room illuminated by fluorescent lights, we no longer hear their hum after a while. If we are at a dinner party with four simultaneous conversations going on and we focus on one conversation, we do not hear the others. Our brains can process only a very small percentage of the information gathered by our senses at any one time. Right now, are you focused on your right big toe? Prior to my mentioning it, my guess is probably not. Unless your toe is hurting, you were probably totally unaware of it. Yet, if you choose to, you can focus your attention on your right big toe. You can also choose to focus on the hum of the fluorescent lights. Our brains are constantly bombarded by sensory input from all five of our senses. It follows that at any given time, our brains can focus on only a relatively small amount of the information gathered by our senses. Were you just thinking about yesterday's breakfast? If we consider all the memories, plans, and other information that our brains contain, it becomes obvious that we can focus on only a miniscule fraction of our brain's content at any one particular time. So normal consciousness is like looking at our finger with one eye through a tube. We are only aware of what is in our limited field of consciousness.

If we are working hard to solve a problem, our focus may be even more pinpoint – like the microscope looking at the wart. That focus really helps if we are studying fine details, but now we have an even more limited field of awareness. (That's usually when your teenage son asks to borrow the car and claims that you said, "Yeah, whatever.") With that skill of focus and concentration, we can solve many a problem. The downside of being so focused, is that when we see a problem, it takes up our whole field of consciousness – like a humongous wart.

To summarize, our brains are only able to process an extremely small fraction of available sensory input at any one time. Problems and danger are particularly good at grabbing the focus of our attention. At times, we focus in even further to address a particular issue. This focusing has several advantages, but it may also compel us to lose perspective, making problems appear much bigger than they really are.

For instance, if one is focused on $1,000 invested in a stock, losing $800 seems devastating. And that's when we need to put down the magnifier and widen our field of vision. Would you sell both your legs or both your eyes for that $800? For a million dollars? For $2 million dollars? If your eyes and legs are functioning normally, your answers are likely: "No, no, and no!" At one of my lectures, an accountant asked if he could sell just one eye for a million dollars. But when you add up all the blessings in life, you wouldn't sell out for all the gold in the world. Neither would the accountant.

One way to regain perspective is to look at the wider picture, and a good way to do that is to remind ourselves of the good things, or blessing in our lives. Remember how you looked at your left index finger through the tube made by your right hand? Listing your blessings is like putting down your right hand and opening both of your eyes. You see a much larger view of the world. If your left index finger symbolized a problem, that problem seems so much smaller now.

*"We can only be said*
*to be alive in those moments*
*when our hearts are conscious*
*of our treasures."*

Thornton Wilder,
playwright and novelist

## GRATITUDE

Several times over the course of a day, look for something for which to be grateful and actually make one of the following statements to yourself:

- "I am grateful to have (blank)."

- "I feel privileged to have (blank) in my life."

- "I am so lucky to have (blank)."

- Or pray, "Thank you for (blank)."

Make these statements with feeling. As you say how grateful you are for a friend or family member in your life, visualize his or her face. Think of different special moments. Think of your health, your ability to see, hear, think and/or feel beauty. Being thankful for the food on your plate (and even the ability to smell and taste good food) will also enhance your mindfulness.

**Practice**

## GRATITUDE JOURNAL

Some people also keep a daily gratitude journal, listing five or 10 new blessings daily. When things are tough, they can review the journal.

*One day a student became very upset, so he went to speak with his teacher. The teacher asked him, "If you had a billion dollars and you lost five dollars, would you be upset?" The student said, "Of course not." The teacher then said to the student, "You are a billionaire." The student then understood that when he considered all he had to be thankful for – his family, friends, and health – he was, in a sense, a billionaire. The next time something went wrong, he thought to himself, "Five bucks," and smiled.*

---

**Relax on the Run**

### FIVE-BUCKS REMINDER

In most instances, if we can take a step back and put a problem in perspective, our stress level decreases markedly. The next time something happens that distresses you, say to yourself, "Five bucks," and remind yourself that you are a billionaire.

---

Now let's really blow your mind: Have you ever wondered about the long shot chance, of all the billions of people on Earth that your parents ever met? Not only that, but in order for you to exist, not only did they need to meet and have sex, but also the sperm that would eventually produce you had to prevail over the other 50 million sperm. Even before that, in order for your parents to be born, your grandparents had to find each other, from all the people on Earth, and that one of 50 million of your grandfathers' sperms had to be the victor. The odds are so high against you ever being born it's unfathomable. Think about how lucky you are to be here. This thought exercise leaves me with a sense of gratitude and awe that I am alive.

Although being the product of a very lucky sperm may fill me with sense of wonder and put a smile on my face, perhaps it doesn't float your gratitude boat. There are other perspectives that are no less awe-inspiring. If you believe in God, isn't it astounding that He chose to give you the miracle of life? Perhaps you believe in reincarnation – there are a billion times more insects than people, so again, you made a very major score. (Don't know about you, but I would certainly rather be human than a dung beetle.) From a variety of different perspectives, even the fact that you exist at all is miraculous.

---

**Relax on the Run**

### REMEMBER THE MIRACLE OF BEING ALIVE

The lucky sperm? God? Not being a dung beetle? If one of those thoughts brings you a smile, remind yourself on a regular basis.

# 8
# Thoughts on Thoughts

Sometimes we handle thoughts like a skilled craftsman – starting with creative dreams and aspirations, leading to realistic goals, and culminating with wonderful plans that can meet our goals. Other times, our use of the tool of thought is more akin to someone hitting his head with a hammer.

We've already reviewed mindfulness as a tool to deal with thoughts. We start by not believing all our thoughts and skillfully and patiently letting some go. It's good to have more than one trick up your sleeve, and in these next three chapters, we will review some other strategies for using our thoughts (rather than being a victim of our thoughts). We will explore the tools of:

- Disputing irrational thoughts

- Reframing

- Restating limiting thoughts

- Focused thinking and creativity

## Disputing Irrational Thoughts
Let's assess your test-taking skills. Pretend you are in school taking a multiple choice test and for the first question there are three possible answers:

A) He always did _____.

B) She never did _____.

C) Sometimes he has done _____.

Since you don't know the question and the blanks could be anything, you can't be sure of the answer. But what's your best guess? I'd argue for answer C. There are few things that are always or never a certain way. When you are talking about someone's behavior the words "always" and "never" are ~~never~~ seldom correct.

So thoughts such as "Life never goes my way" or "I can't do anything right" would be incorrect. These are examples of what psychologists call irrational beliefs or cognitive distortions. And more often than not, it's not the events alone that cause the stress. It's not even the thoughts alone that cause the stress. The stress often emanates from the belief in the irrational thoughts.

Consider this scenario: Your boss yells and you have a series of thoughts: "I can't do anything right ... I'll probably get fired ... I'll never get another job ... He probably thinks I'm a total failure." Will you become extremely stressed?

That depends on your next step:

   a. You believe all those thoughts and dwell
      on them. This will lead to a dump truck full
      of stress.

   b. You resist the thoughts: "I just need a clear
      mind. Why am I bothered by so many irratio-
      nal thoughts?" Again, your level of relaxation
      just took a nosedive.

   c. You notice the thoughts and let them go –
      without believing them, but without taking
      the effort to dispute them. Over the past

chapters, we've reviewed this as an effective option to decrease your stress.

d. You dispute the irrational thoughts. "I made one mistake. That does not mean I do everything wrong." "I've done most of my work correctly, and I doubt that I'd get fired for doing one thing wrong"; "If I did get fired, it might be a little difficult, but I'd find another job"; "He just yelled at me today. Maybe he is having a bad day. I know that when I yell at somebody, it has more to do with my inner frustration than anything else." Disputing these types of irrational beliefs usually decreases stress, anger, frustration, and sadness.

If you want to effectively deal with stress, depending on the circumstances, you may choose either option c (just let the thoughts go) or option d (dispute irrational thoughts).

Let's look at the most common types of *irrational beliefs* that hamper relaxation:

We've already discussed the always/never overgeneralization type irrational beliefs.

Let's discuss some others:

Remember Eeyore? He was the old gray donkey that hung out with Winnie the Pooh. If you can imagine Eeyore saying something, then it's likely an irrational belief.

Certainly you could imagine Eeyore saying, "Nothing ever goes right." If something did go well, Eeyore would likely minimize its importance. Or he would play the pessimistic fortune teller, saying, "It will probably never happen again."

Couldn't you picture Eeyore doing a little mind reading: "Owl didn't say 'hello'. I'm sure he doesn't like me." He doesn't consider that Owl may have been preoccupied with his problems.

The grand prize for the cognitive distortion creating the most stress goes to catastrophizing. A relatively small matter goes wrong and you say phrases such as: "This is a nightmare, it is horrible, it is a catastrophe." And lo and behold, by thinking like Eeyore, you're stressed.

If you lose $50 and say that it was horrifying, I would suggest that most likely, it is not horrifying, but you are "Eeyorifying." (From the Dr. Winner Made-Up Word Dictionary, Page 137: Eeyorify: (verb) to believe irrational thoughts – like Eeyore.)

One remedy, as mentioned earlier, is to dispute those thoughts. Instead of "this is a nightmare," use the likely more accurate phrase, "this is unfortunate."

---

**Relax on the Run**

## IRRATIONAL THOUGHTS

Recognize irrational thoughts and either dispute them or just let them go.

---

When first learning to recognize cognitive distortions, it can help to chart them on paper. Just writing down an irrational belief often allows you to see how truly irrational it is. Here is an example:

| Situation | Emotions | Auto-matic Thoughts | Dispute (Ratioinal Response) |
|---|---|---|---|
| Your boss yells at you. | Sadness, anger | "I can't do anything right." | "I did one thing wrong, but I've done a lot right." |
| Frustration | "He prob-ably thinks that I'm a total fail-ure." | "He had a short fuse today." | "I can't assume that he thinks poorly of me." |

*Denise worked setting up displays at a store. On one occasion, Denise spent an entire day setting up a particular display exactly as instructed. After all that work, her boss changed her mind about what she wanted. Denise was very upset. She found herself thinking, "This is horrible! I can't believe this happened." When she realized that she was catastrophizing, she corrected herself in a way that was much closer to the truth: "It's inconvenient that I will have to set up a new display." Once she realized that the situation was not the end of the world, she felt much better and stopped working herself into a frenzy.*

In time, you will automatically recognize cognitive distortions and quickly act to dispel them.

# 9

# Reframing

In 1897, Jerome Monroe Smucker started what would become an $8.6 billion dollar company. I would imagine that Jerome was proud of his name on the fruit spreads. Can you imagine an advertising executive first suggesting the slogan "With a name like Smucker's, it has to be good"? Jerome Smucker or his son must have been all, "What's wrong with our name? Get out of our office and stay out!" Even better was when "Saturday Night Live" made a spoof of the Smucker's commercials – something like: "With a name like Monkey Brains, it has to be good!" Unless it had a reputation of being the fruit spread of the angels, Monkey Brain jam would not be my pick. When I discussed this with one of my 11-year-old twin sons, he exclaimed, "I would totally buy a jam called Monkey Brains!" Would he actually eat a monkey's brains – no way! But to his mind, the name was absolutely boss.

So is Smucker's a good or bad name? Is Monkey Brains a good or bad name? It all depends on your viewpoint. And, good for us, we can change our viewpoint to suit the circumstances.

Reframing involves assuming a new view of a given set of circumstances. By changing your interpretation, you change your stress response. Initially, you might view a difficult task as an objectionable chore. By reframing, you can view the task as an enjoyable challenge.

> **"We are continually faced by great opportunities brilliantly disguised as insoluble problems."**
>
> Lee Iacocca,
> past CEO of Ford and Chyrsler

> **"The pessimist sees difficulty in every opportunity. The optimist sees opportunity in every difficulty."**
>
> Winston Churchill

Thomas Edison worked long, hard hours and failed in many of his attempts to invent the incandescent light bulb. If his response to his initially unsuccessful efforts was, "I'm a loser. I can't do anything right," we might all still be in the dark. (And I probably wouldn't include his quotation.) But instead, Edison said, "I am not discouraged, because every wrong attempt discarded is another step forward."

Acute lymphoblastic leukemia (ALL) used to be a uniformly fatal illness, and researchers were frustrated in their attempts to help children with this devastating disease. In the early 1940s, folic acid was first synthesized. Since doctors were desperate to find a treatment for ALL, Dr. Sidney Farber tried giving folic acid to children with the illness. Unfortunately, giving folic acid to those children was exactly the wrong thing to do – the children died more quickly.

When faced with a move that made the situation worse, did Dr. Farber just give up? No. Instead, he wondered, if the children died more quickly with folic acid, what would happen if the children were given a drug that inhibited the action of folic acid? What, indeed! The children lived longer, and thus, in 1947, a folic acid inhibitor, aminopterin, became the first major breakthrough in the fight against childhood leukemia. What had been a uniformly fatal disease that took so many young lives, now has a cure rate of about 90 percent.

How many times have we berated ourselves for not doing something correctly, or sometimes even for not doing something perfectly? Instead of interpreting an effort as a failure, it's much more productive to reframe an unsuccessful effort as an opportunity to learn. The nature of science is to see what didn't work and then change it up. And the same goes for almost any other endeavor. That's how society advances. When we are willing to learn, there is no more effective teacher than our errors.

---

**Relax on the Run**

### WHEN YOU DON'T SUCCEED

When you don't succeed, reframe it as an opportunity to learn.

---

Few things are more stressful than having someone be rude to you. Whether it's at the bank or Aunt Martha's house, it can send your blood pressure right through the roof. But a little reflection can change all that.

Over the years, in my stress management classes, I've asked several thousand people two simple questions:

1. "Who here has ever been rude?" Typically, everyone in the audience raises their hands.

2. Next I ask: "When you have been rude, is it usually when you are happy and feeling your best?" And there are no hands in the air.

Thousands of people giving the exact same answers to these two questions provide overwhelming evidence for a simple conclusion. It reveals an often ignored principle; yet on reflection, it is an obvious truth – when people act rude, they are probably suffering. Bear this in mind when an acquaintance is rude. Instead of immediately reacting with anger, realize that he or she may not be doing well. Did the bank teller's wife just file for divorce? Did your boss just find out about her sister's breast cancer?

On a daily basis we communicate with people we don't know well, and therefore, know very little about what is going on in their lives and their minds. Even with close friends and family, we can't know all of the issues that may be troubling them. If people are rude, almost undoubtedly they are unhappy. At times, it may be helpful to ask if something is bothering them. Other times, it might only inflame the situation. In either case, it decreases your own stress and hostility to appreciate that the surface rudeness probably stems from a deeper suffering that has little to do with you.

When dealing with rude people, it pays to learn from the experts – people who, through their job, must routinely interact with annoyed folks. For instance, one of the responsibilities of an emergency room doctor is to call other doctors at 2 a.m., wake them up, and persuade them to come into the hospital to admit a patient. In other words, the ER doc might not be catching these folks at their most cheery time. But it gets much worse: ER physicians routinely deal with barrages of obscene-laden language delivered by drunk and psychotic patients. How does an ER doctor deal with all that verbal abuse?

One ER doctor said that the best training for this was not from medical school or from residency – instead, it came from his time before medical school when he worked as a waiter. Then, as customers complained, "The ice is too cold" or "The water is too wet," he learned to cheerfully reply, "Sorry, sir; I'll take care of that right away." He learned not to take rude behavior personally – instead of being insulted, he reflexively reframed such behavior as evidence of another's suffering.

What about the people who seem to be rude most of the time? Well, perhaps they are unhappy most of the time. Perhaps they are clinically depressed or are in chronic pain. Also, remember that rudeness may simply spring from a difference in communication styles. For instance, a fast-talking person may seem rude to someone not accustomed to such brusqueness.

Communication is such a tricky combination of language, jargon, slang, gestures, and tone and volume of voice that it's a wonder we can ever understand each other at all.

In summary, if someone is rude, he or she is most likely suffering, and the uncommon exceptions to that rule usually involve some sort of miscommunication. Either way, a little understanding and reframing are routinely the right remedy to rudeness.

*I once called a business associate and a woman answered the telephone in a shockingly rude manner. She asked, "Why the (blank) are you calling again?" I was stunned but asked to speak with my associate. She refused to take a message or to give me another way to reach him. I was tempted to give her some of her own rude medicine. Instead, I told myself that she must be having a really, really bad day, that her rudeness had nothing to do with me, and that there was no way I could fix the situation. I politely ended the call. When I spoke to my associate later, I learned that the woman was his 82-year-old mother. She was filling in and answering the phones and was extremely stressed. This information made her behavior much more understandable. I was certainly glad that I had chosen to reframe the situation – for my sake and hers.*

**Relax on the Run**

## WHEN PEOPLE ARE RUDE

When someone is rude ... remember that most likely they are suffering in one way or another. Also consider that there may be a miscommunication.

A woman in one of my classes was a supervisor for a group of receptionists. The receptionists were barraged daily with customer complaints. The supervisor advised that they look at each complaint as an opportunity to make a positive difference in someone's life.

---

## HEARING COMPLAINTS

Hearing complaints can be reframed as a chance to make a positive difference in someone's life. Sometimes you might be able to solve a problem or at least help figure out a plan of action. Other times, just empathetically listening and/or helping someone reframe a situation can help.

---

Another woman supervised a staff who answered the phones at a psychiatric hospital. The staff received many rude calls and were bothered by them, so the supervisor decided to start a contest. The person who received the rudest call of the week would win a prize. This brilliant bit of reframing transformed each nasty, stress-inducing call into an opportunity for fun. The staff was almost happy to get the rude calls. You can imagine them joyfully asking, "You called me a what? How do you spell that?" It didn't take much of a prize to help them gain some new perspective.

---

## MAKE A CONTEST

If there is a group stressor, can you use some creativity to come up with a contest?

---

Some people become annoyed if they have to do some un-expected walking. They could reframe the situation and be thankful for the opportunity to exercise. There is nothing more ironic than people fighting to park as close as possible to the entrance of their health club so they can rush inside and work out on a treadmill.

---

**Relax on the Run**

## AN EXTRA WALK

An extra walk is an opportunity for more exercise.

---

Imagine that you are in a grocery store. You pick the shortest checkout line because you are in a rush. However, as the line next to you moves like a greyhound, yours bogs down like a turtle in mud. You find yourself fuming that it is your fate to always pick the slowest line. You get annoyed as you watch the customer in front of you, who starts paying with a credit card but then changes his mind and decides that paying with a check would be better. Then he remembers the 12 coupons in his pocket. So the cashier starts over and the customer writes a new check. Your blood pressure continues to rise. How would you reframe this situation?

In these busy times, many of us rush from one task to another. We seldom have free time. I would reframe this wait at the grocery store as just that. I'd view it as an opportunity to focus on my breathing, reflect on my plans, maybe to list those aspects of my life for which I'm grateful. I might catch up on checking emails on my phone. I might even chat with another person in line or indulge in the opportunity to flip through a magazine I wouldn't normally buy. (You know, the magazines that say things like George Clooney is really an alien from planet Pluto – which is totally absurd since Pluto is no longer a planet.)

Free time. How many of us get enough? I know plenty of people who are stressed out over their lack of free time. Yet, ironically, in a typical week we find ourselves waiting through a variety of activities and getting stressed out about that. Whether you're put on hold while calling an office, standing in line at the Department of Motor Vehicles, at the bank, or stuck in a traffic jam, it is key to be able to reframe these waits as opportunities to take a break from your busy day. Once you do this, potential times of stress become times to indulge yourself and relax.

*Sally had an enlargement in her cheek that was thought to be a tumor. She was scheduled for an MRI scan and was terrified of the prospect of lying still in a tube for 40 minutes while being scanned. She had worked herself into a frenzy and was about to ask her doctor for some Valium when she decided to reframe the situation instead. She reminded herself that she was always busy, doing one thing or another. She never had time to sit and reflect about the situations and people in her life for which she was grateful. The MRI scan could be a special time of solitude when no one would interrupt her. These thoughts gave a new meaning to the scan and soothed her anxiety. The tumor turned out to be benign. Since then, whenever Sally is in a traffic jam or similar circumstance, she reminds herself to appreciate her solitude and the opportunity to reflect on her life.*

## WAITING

Times to wait can be reframed as an opportunity to take a break from your busy day.

## Physical and Emotional Pain

Let's think about emotional and physical pain in another way. A weightlifter's muscles really hurt during and after a workout. If, out of the blue, your biceps started aching like that, you would knock on a doctor's door without delay. However, the weightlifter doesn't visit a doctor. He may even enjoy the pain. Why? To him, the pain has a meaning. It signifies that his muscles are growing and getting stronger. It reminds him that he's working hard. If the pain had no meaning, it would be something to be avoided. Childbirth is an example of intense pain that becomes part of a joyous experience because of its context: The pain is a necessary part of a wonderful event.

We have all gone through painful experiences, and when we can find meaning in those experiences, it helps to decrease our suffering. Perhaps you are distressed about your physical condition and don't like the way you look and feel. You can dwell on this distress, or you can use that feeling to motivate you to start an exercise program. Once you make that decision, it helps alleviate your suffering. The pain had a purpose. It was there not to make you miserable, but to stimulate you to take action and make changes.

Perhaps you suffer from a painful condition, such as rheumatoid arthritis. Even in this situation, you can choose to dwell on the stress and pain, or you can decide that your condition challenges you to find the best medical and behavioral treatments. Not only that, the pain might have further meaning if you start a support group to help others, or if you decide to help the local Arthritis Foundation. It may seem difficult, and pain is never fun, but the way you choose to view it can go a long way toward making it bearable.

I would prefer it if neither my family nor I ever had any serious medical problems. However, my luck in that regard has not been perfect. Sooner or later, we all will see pain and illness in our families. It slightly decreases my pain to find meaning in the fact that any pain I have experienced increases my empathy for other people. It makes me a better physician, communicator, and human being. In this regard, I have learned more as a patient or a family member of a patient than I have in most of my medical school classes.

*When our twins were 8 months old, my wife and I planned a trip to visit relatives. About an hour into the trip, we had a blowout on the freeway. That's right, our right rear tire shredded with people going 70 miles an hour all around us. My wife very understandably said, "This is a nightmare!" It was a bad situation, but catastrophizing would not make it better. So I said, "This is definitely not ideal, but we'll manage." I was able to slowly drive onto the shoulder and get to a small road that was much less busy.*

*As my wife watched the boys, I emptied the back of the station wagon (which had been carefully packed to the brim) to get to the spare and then proceeded to change the tire. Together, my wife and I reframed the situation and agreed that it had been lucky that the flat had happened while we were together (as opposed to her being alone with the boys); that it had happened during the daytime; that it had not been raining; and that there had been a small street just a half mile up the road where we could much more safely stop than if we had been stuck on the shoulder of the freeway.*

---

**Relax on the Run**

### FINDING THE MEANING IN PAIN

It can be challenging to find a silver lining in difficult circumstances, emotional and/or physical pain. However, finding some meaning in the pain, may decrease your suffering. Try asking yourself: Did the pain or can the pain:

- motivate you toward a goal or a positive life change?

- result in growing closer to family and/or old friends?

- result in developing new relationships?

- make you wiser in any way?

- make you more resilient?

- make you more empathetic?

---

**Optional Audio Exercise:** Letting Go and Reframing Exercise available at www.stressremedy.com

# 10

# More Fun with Thoughts and Imagination

## Visualization

If you are likely to encounter a particular stressful event, it may help to visuaulize yourself using the techniques you have learned to effectively deal with the stress. The following guided exercise is a good way to practice for such events.

**Practice**

### VISUALIZE PROBLEMS AND SOLUTIONS

If you know you may encounter a stressful situation, can you visualize a better way of handling it – perhaps using reframing, mindfulness, keeping things in perspective and/or disputing irrational beliefs.

Are you having trouble figuring out a way to deal with or finding a new way to look at a particularly stressful situation? In *A Path with a Heart*, Jack Kornfield describes a great visualization you can use to help:

**Practice**

## WISE VISITOR VISUALIZATION

Close your eyes and imagine you are in the midst of the situation. Imagine the problem playing out the way it normally does, and then at the peak of the stress, there is a knock at the door. When you answer the door, you see the wisest, most compassionate person you can imagine. It could be a person you know personally, or it could be a religious figure, philosopher or prophet: Buddha, Jesus, Socrates, Santa, Whoopi Goldberg — whomever you'd most like to see at that moment. That person offers to take over your body for a few minutes and handles the situation. Observe how he or she handle it. What can you learn? After she gives you back your body, imagine she gives you a piece of advice. What might she say? As you reflect on the advice, realize that it was you who had the wisdom and handled the situation all along.

## Affirmations

We talked of reminders to be mindful. At times, other reminders are useful.

*Stan would get nervous at his singing auditions. Despite being well prepared, he would question if he picked the wrong song or if he was ill-prepared. Prior to his auditions, Stan would remind himself, "I am prepared; I am confident; I'll do great." These brief reminders improved Stan's auditions.*

At the end of a lecture, a physician commented that he awoke every day looking forward to his day at the office. He felt privileged to work with his patients. It was a moving comment and mirrored how I thought of my work. However, at some points during the day, perhaps as I was running late and anticipated that my next patient would have complicated issues, I'd feel just a bit of dread. I was ready for the day to be over and I was ready for the day to be over so I could just relax at home. This was the time when it was useful to remind myself, "I am privileged to have a wonderful job – a job in which I am able to get to know and care for people." This affirmation gave me the energy and enthusiasm to enjoy the rest of my day.

---

**Relax on the Run**

**AFFIRMATION**

A short, true positive phrase can, at times, reduce stress and increase confidence.

---

## Internal versus External Locus of Control

*"The best years of your life are the ones in which you decide your problems are your own. You do not blame them on your mother, the ecology or the president. You realize that you control your own destiny."*

Albert Elllis, psychologist who developed rational emotive behavior therapy

*"Things turn out best for the people who make the best of the way things turn out."*

John Wooden, basketball coach

In the early 1970s, W. Mitchell was in a motorcycle accident and suffered a severe burn affecting 65 percent of his body, including his face and hands. Despite this severe injury, he co-founded a company that was later valued at 65 million dollars. Four years after the first accident, he had a second accident, which left him paraplegic. Despite that injury, he became the mayor of a small town in Colorado and successfully campaigned to stop the destruction of a mountain. At first, Mitchell found his wheelchair a terrible prison, that kept him from doing the things he wanted. Later, he reframed his situation, and the wheelchair became a magical apparatus that helped him travel throughout the world. He says that, before the accidents, he "could do 9,000 things; after the accident 8,000 things." He chose to celebrate the 8,000 things he could do, rather than dwell on the 1,000 things he couldn't. His philosophy is embodied in the title of his book: *It's Not What Happens to You. It's What You Do About It.*

Which begs the question: What determines your happiness? What happens to you or what you do about it? Cognitive psychologists discuss this issue in terms of "locus of control." Having an "external locus of control" means thinking that your happiness and satisfaction depend primarily on the external environment. In contrast, having an "internal locus of control" means thinking that most of your happiness and satisfaction depend on the choices that you make and the way you view life. In short, do you look for your happiness from within or without? A stressed person, with an internal locus of control, would be more solution-oriented, thinking for instance, about how he might view the situation differently, be more mindful, or change the situation. It's no surprise to learn that people with an internal locus of control tend to handle stress better than people with an external one. One of the purposes of this book is to give you a greater internal locus of control.

To change one's locus of control, we should examine the importance of language, whether spoken by our lips or just echoing in our heads. the words we use can make a big difference in determining our locus of control. For instance, if I say, "He made me angry," I give all the responsibility for my anger to "him." I lose control over my own state of mind.

Think about these two phrases:

1. "I got angry, because she left the top off the toothpaste."

2. "She left the top off the toothpaste and I got angry."

In the first sentence, I had no choice but to be angry. That anger was the inevitable response to the action. The second sentence acknowledges that there were other options. There was still a connection between the action and the emotion, but the choice was mine. I could have thought it was funny and laughed. I could have been sad, or not cared. By restating the thought in a different way, I gave myself a choice in how I responded. This might sound insignificant, but the next time you think someone made you feel a certain way, try correcting yourself. You may be surprised by the subsequent change in your attitude.

---

**Relax on the Run**

### RESTATE EXTERNAL LOCUS
### OF CONTROL STATEMENTS

When you say, "I'm angry because of blank" or "He made me angry," try restating the phrase "Blank happened and I got angry."

See if you feel any different.

---

We limit ourselves with language in other ways. First thing one beautiful morning, when one of my sons was 6 years old, he spilled a drink. Then out of his mouth comes, "I'm having a bad day." I had to chuckle (very quietly) to myself, since that phrase sounded a bit funny coming from a 6-year-old. But how often, like my son, do we give ourselves self-fulfilling prophecies? One tiny thing goes wrong and – Bam! – we think, "I'm having a bad day." And then, sure enough, we do have a bad day.

Consider the statements "I can't do math" and "Every time my boss criticizes me, I get very upset." Compare them with "In the past, I have had trouble with math" and "In the past, when my boss criticized me, I would get very upset." As you can see, the latter statements leave open your options for how to act in the future. They leave control, and responsibility, squarely on your shoulders. And just knowing that you have that internal locus of control goes a long way toward reducing stress and cultivating happiness.

Do you limit yourself with your thoughts in still other ways? Imagine a woman with four young children saying to herself, "I can't be happy in a disorganized house." Certainly, she may feel better if her house were organized and organizing your house is a worthy goal (a stress-reducer in its own right). However, with four young children, chances are, at any given time, her house will not be perfectly organized. She has, therefore, limited herself to being unhappy much of the time. If you limit yourself to being happy only in very specific circumstances, you have lost a lot of potentially wonderful moments.

---

**Relax on the Run**

### RESTATE LIMITATIONS

Notice if, through thought or spoken word, you've unnecessarily limited yourself. If so, restate the thought. For instance, you might say, "In the past...," thus leaving open the possibility of future changes.

---

Setting an intention can also help.

---

**Relax on the Run**

### SETTING AN INTENTION FOR THE DAY

Perhaps after listing your blessings or giving thanks, as you start your day, say to yourself a statement such as "May I live today wisely and joyously." If you like, substitute other words for "wisely" and "joyously," such as lovingly, mindfully, kindly, etc.

---

When you say words like this in the morning, likely they will come to mind later in the day. And when they do so, it will be a reminder that at every moment, no matter what the circumstances, your attitude is your choice, so you might as well live wisely, lovingly, and kindly.

Developing an internal locus of control allows you to use yet another type of reframing. By now, you have likely realized that the way you view a situation and the way you train your mind largely determine your stress level. Therefore, every hardship, every time you become irritated can be seen as an opportunity to train your mind and to grow. Each challenge you meet makes you more prepared for the next one.

> *Rosalyn had spent many hours while on vacation working on her first oil painting. Painting was a highlight of her trip, and she looked forward to hanging the framed artwork in her living room. Unfortunately, it was destroyed on the plane on the way home. Initially, she was understandably distressed.*
>
> *Rosalyn used several of the techniques described in this and the previous chapter to deal with her stress. She disputed irrational beliefs about the ruined artwork. Instead of "The vacation is ruined," she thought, "This is unfortunate." Instead of "How dumb of me not to get a box to protect the painting," she thought, "Now I know to protect my next painting with a box before I travel."*

*She also reframed the situation. The most import-
ant part of this painting was the fun she had had
working on it. She was now motivated to pursue
a wonderful new hobby. That motivation was still
unblemished.*

*Rosalyn also thought of Buddhist monks spend-
ing several weeks making an intricate design out
of sand. When the beautiful design is finished, it
is appreciated. Then it is destroyed and the sand
is poured into the ocean. The design is used as an
example of life's impermanence. Rosalyn took a
cue from the monks and used her disappointment
as an opportunity to train her mind. By learning
to deal with this situation effectively, she would
be better prepared for life's future challenges. She
better honed her skills in disputing irrational
beliefs, in reframing, and in letting go of thoughts
of how life should be. Instead, she focused on enjoying life as it is – like the scenic drive at the end of
the vacation.*

Thoughts can subconsciously confine you to a certain
view of reality. However, when you take a step back, you
will recognize that the walls that formed that reality were
just thoughts. You can renovate those mental walls into
something more comfortable. You can see that, instead
of being overwhelmed, you had a thought that you were
overwhelmed. Instead of the traffic making you angry,
you had a thought that the traffic made you angry. Taking
this step back allows you to let certain thoughts go in
order to enjoy the present moment. You may also dispute
or reframe thoughts to better manage your stress.

# 11

# Rushing 'round the Clock

Waiting in line at the counter, mouth full of potato chips that he had not yet bought, crumbs spurting out the sides of his mouth with every word, left index finger pointing to an oversize sandwich, the man rushed to get out the words: "I'll have an extra-large one of those with everything on it!" The fast food wasn't fast enough. Do you ever see at least a little bit of that Not-Fast-Enough-Food (NFEF) guy in yourself? If not in line at a fast food place, somewhere else? I sure do. There are times when instead of relaxing in the moment, I have this drive to quench my hunger. Sometimes, like NFEF guy, there is a hunger for food and other times it may be a hunger to get work done or hunger to have my back feel better.

There's nothing at all wrong with moving fast. I'm not going to tell Michael Phelps, "You really need to slow down in the pool." There are very appropriate times to move fast. The problem is when we can't slow down. The challenge is in learning to not feel constantly driven; not having a constant sense of urgency.

If you're having a blast as you race around the track of life – cool! However, if you're racing around the track because you feel like a rabid dog is chasing you – not so cool.

Buddhists use the metaphor of "hungry ghosts" to illustrate a non-stop drive to satisfy desire. The hungry ghosts have tiny mouths and throats, but have huge stomachs; thus, their hunger can never be satisfied. Psychologist Carl Rogers called this sense of being driven Deficiency, or D motivation.

Compare this to the dancer, musician or artist who does their work with a sense of play and enjoyment. They have what Carl Rogers termed Being, or B motivation. Do you want to live your life with a sense of being compulsively driven? Might you accomplish the same tasks with relaxation instead of urgency? With enjoyment instead of anxiety?

According to a popular story, Meyer Friedman and Ray H. Rosenman noticed that their waiting-room chairs were wearing out way too fast. Looking into the room, they did not find a group of patients with sandpaper on their butts. Instead, they noticed a very impatient, anxious group of people sitting almost on the front edges of their chairs. They said people with this type behavior had what they termed to be a "Type A personality." If Drs. Friedman and Rosenman were proctologists, they may have assumed that this personality style was associated with an elevated risk of hemorrhoids. However, since they were cardiologists, they assumed Type A personality was linked to heart disease.

While people with "Type B personalities" tend to be more mellow and laid back, those with Type A personalities continuously struggle to accomplish more and more. They have a sense of time urgency, often when there is no real reason to rush. The urgency includes talking very quickly and finishing others' sentences, driving and eating fast, and multitasking.

Type A people tend to be more aggressive and hostile. Although there has been some controversy about the effect of Type A behavior on heart disease, excessive anger and hostility have been clearly shown to be related to heart disease in several studies. One study followed 1,305 men for seven years. The men with the greatest levels of anger had 2.66 times the risk of developing a heart problem. Additionally, time urgency, impatience, and hostility are associated with a significant increase in the long-term risk of high blood pressure.

For convenience and fun, let's abbreviate the quality of having a Type A personality as "Type A-ness" or "A-ness". And, in those times when you're driven to race around like a cheetah – then you've got major A-ness! And nobody wants that. In fact, your A-ness (not to be confused with Uranus) will interfere with your ability to relax and enjoy life. The aggravation, impatience, anger, and irritation associated with A-ness are not the most conducive to great relationships, so people with major A-ness often get the reputation of being a real pain in the ... neck.

People with a Type A personality are often under the impression that this hurry sickness will improve the proficiency. However, often, by rushing around they get lost in detail – as the saying goes, they lose sight of the forest for the trees. And thereby, they actually decrease proficiency and productivity.

*Cindy worked in a retail store. Like many people in the retail business, she was often rushed for time. One day, a demanding customer was taking a long time at the store. Instead of spending an extra two minutes addressing this person's concerns, Cindy became impatient. By cutting her time with this customer short, she saved those two minutes. However, later that day, she remembered what she'd done and it bothered her. She spent some time justifying her actions to herself, then spent some more time feeling bad and wondering if she had been rude.*

*The next day, the customer complained to Cindy's supervisor. Cindy then had to spend an extra 30 minutes writing a response to his complaint. Cindy might not have done anything technically wrong, but in the long run she saved only two minutes by rushing a conversation with the customer, and those two minutes ultimately cost her much more time feeling stressed about the interaction and responding to the complaint.*

The book *The House of God* is a sarcastic novel that looks at the difficult life of medical residents in the 1970s. In the book, experienced residents teach new residents certain "laws" of residency. One of the laws had to do with how one should act in dealing with a cardiac arrest (when a patient's heart stops): "At a cardiac arrest, the first procedure is to take your own pulse." For someone who has never "run a code" (i.e., directed the staff in caring for someone having a cardiac arrest), this law probably seems like a joke in poor taste. Only those of us who have run a code understand it.

When someone's heart has stopped, there is the temptation to frantically bounce around like a ping-pong ball in an earthquake. When you are frantic in a code, you are inefficient and more likely to make a mistake – you're all discombobulated! (As opposed to "combobulated"? Should be a word if it's not, as in: "Nancy is so calm and combobulated.")

Even when someone's heart stops, it can be much more effective for a doctor to take two or three seconds and one mindful diaphragmatic breath before acting. That way, the doctor can remember his or her training and act efficiently and thoughtfully. I wouldn't spend an entire minute taking my own pulse, but a couple of seconds to take that diaphragmatic breath could help save a life.

I know that most of you aren't in the position of having to regularly respond to cardiac arrests. But consider this: Not many emergencies are more pressing than someone's heart stopping; yet, even then, it makes sense to take one diaphragmatic breath before acting. If you need to push someone off the train tracks before a train hits him, you might not have those two seconds. For almost all other "personal emergencies," you can and should spare at least that amount of time.

*In our frantic lives, we sometimes have to remind ourselves that we're not in the middle of an emergency. In the 1990s, I occasionally worked weekend shifts as a doctor in an understaffed urgent care center. Since there were no scheduled appointments, patient waiting times were often long. One Sunday, an unusually large number of patients had to be seen, and the wait was well over two hours. I found myself exhibiting Type A behavior – frequently interrupting patients and rushing them along. Suddenly I realized that no one was dying.*

*I decided that on the following Monday, I would advise the administration that we needed more staff on weekends. But in the meantime, I needed a strategy for the current weekend. My Type A strategy of rushing and interrupting patients was saving only a few minutes, at best. And it was unfair to the patients. If someone had already waited two hours, the last thing he or she needed was a doctor who interrupted every other sentence.*

*Instead, I decided to shift my perspective and give each patient a more considered interaction with me. Seeing a doctor who listened empathetically would certainly be worth an additional 10-minute wait to these patients. On that long day, I saw more than 40 patients. However, I was not stressed, and the patients did seem more appreciative, despite their wait, since their problems were carefully and considerately addressed.*

If you rush through the workday at a harried pace, interrupting people and trying to do several projects at once just to get home 30 minutes earlier, it is probably not worth the additional stress. Although it is important to have time at home, it is better to enjoy working an 8 1/2-hour day than to spend an 8-hour day in distress.

**"Enjoy the little things, for one day you may look back and realize they were the big things."**

Robert Brault, author

People with a Type A personality often worry about wasting time, but what is the real waste of time? Does wasting time mean that you don't work every second of the day? I would argue that life is too short to squander by being compulsively driven. The real waste of time is not enjoying this moment.

Some researchers feel that a major factor in the development of the type A personality style is low self-esteem and a continuing need to prove oneself. Low self-esteem cannot be improved by the frantic pursuit of material objects or achievements. It is important to have an inherent sense of self-worth. Most people in my classes say that they are willing to believe that all of us have inherent worth, independent of any accomplishments. If you have a thought otherwise, remember it is just a thought that can be let go, and then return to enjoy the next breath. If it surfaces again, gently let it go again.

> *"No one can make you feel inferior without your consent."*
>
> Eleanor Roosevelt

---

**Relax on the Run**

## NOTICE WHEN YOU FEEL AN UNDUE SENSE OF URGENCY

When you notice this, take a mindful breath and perhaps relax your body, or do the valet pose discussed in Chapter 1, or do another brief mindfulness exercise. Resume your activity in a more relaxed fashion.

## LIFESTYLE TIPS

## WHEN DO I RUSH?

Are there times when you typically rush unnecessarily? List some of these times, then consider solutions. Should you wake up a little earlier so you don't have to rush? Are you overscheduled? Or can you just practice taking your time without any of these external changes?

1. _____

2. _____

3. _____

4. _____

5. _____

## Practice

## SLOW-MOTION LIVING

On occasion, when you have a little more time, try setting aside that time to practice moving very slowly. Do a walking meditation, and bring your awareness to the sensations in your legs and feet. As you reach to open a door, notice your arm reaching. You might even note to yourself, "Reaching." As you turn the doorknob, notice your hand turning the doorknob. Of course, it is not practical to always move this slowly. Perhaps, for the few minutes after a sitting meditation, you can try moving slowly and mindfully. If you are going on a vacation or retreat, maybe you can spend more time moving at a slow, purposeful pace. Practicing this type of mindfulness, in slow motion, can carry over as you resume a more normal pace.

# 12

# Balance and Time

It was first introduced in the 1960s: a colorful, inflatable vinyl clown, weighted at the bottom with sand. For us kids, the object was to punch the clown, just to have it pop right back up. Sure they look harmless enough, but they were almost like the legendary hydra – as Hercules cut off one the hydra's heads, two new huge poison-spewing heads would grow back. When you punched the clown, he'd come back with vengeance.

I might be slightly overstating the power of the blow-up Bozo, but he was resilient. Sure, a pin would quickly do him in, but the way he could come back after a 6-year-old punched him made Muhammed Ali's Rope-A-Dope look amateurish. And why did he did he keep popping back up? It was all about the balance. Balance helps make us resilient.

The inflato-clown's balance came from a low center of gravity. Our balance comes from wisely investing our time and effort into various areas of our lives: friends, family, work, hobbies, exercise, etc. If you spend the vast majority of your time and effort focused just on your job, what happens when something goes wrong at the workplace? You might have trouble popping right back up.

Put another way: If you put all your eggs in one basket and there's a mishap, don't be surprised by the huge sloppy omelet of a mess on the ground. Better you should have a little scrambled eggs with lox on one plate, a little egg salad sandwich on a second, an egg over hard on the third plate, and a plain hardboiled egg on the fourth. You drop the hardboiled egg – no big deal – just feed it to the dog, and move on. You've got plenty left to eat and only a small mess.

Divide your time and effort wisely between family life, friends, work life, hobbies and exercise. For families with young children, likely much of your time will be with the whole family, but it also makes sense to put some time and effort into your relationship with your spouse.

"Sure," you say, "I'll have more of a balance later." There are times that makes sense – perhaps you need a short burst of extra effort as you finish a project. If you're not careful, however, postponing a balanced life can be treacherous slope.

As you get older, does time seem to move slower or faster? If you're like me, 20 minutes of sitting in seventh grade social studies seemed to take a year. Yet now, at times, a year seems to take 20 minutes. Don't let your life get away from you.

*Bonnie's parents were well-off financially, and growing up she had become accustomed to a relatively costly lifestyle. She and her husband worked hard to continue that lifestyle, and before she knew it, she was working four jobs. Although none of the jobs was full time, the combination was much more than full time. After taking my stress management class, she started to realize that her lifestyle was costing her more than just money. Her stress was markedly reduced when she made some changes, including selling her expensive car and quitting two of her jobs.*

> **"Why should we be in such desperate haste to succeed, and in such desperate enterprises? If a man does not keep pace with his companions, perhaps it is because he hears a different drummer."**
>
> Henry David Thoreau
> American author, poet, and philosopher

---

**LIFESTYLE TIPS**

### BALANCE

Take some time to reflect on whether your life is out of balance. If so, write down some general goals and specific plans to bring more balance to your life.

---

## Social Support

If you chat with a hospice worker and ask about people's most common regrets on their deathbeds, it's almost never, "I wish I had spent more time working." It's commonly: "I wish I had spent more time with my family and/or friends." What type of friendships are important for mental and physical health? One hint: Hospice patients are usually not pining away wishing they had more Facebook or Instagram friends. Social websites might enhance communication between close friends, but having the most "friends," virtual or otherwise, does not make the big difference in mental or physical health.

On the other hand, having even a few close friends, relationships in which people really care and support each other – that does make the difference. Physical benefits of a good social support system range from an increased resistance to colds to a lower incidence of heart disease. Certainly, a network of good friends can improve one's emotional health.

Social support may come from family, old schoolmates or relatively new acquaintances. Devote enough time to nurture your old relationships and don't let small grievances ruin a good friendship. Take the time to reconnect, even if it is with a brief chat over the phone.

Be open to new connections. Perhaps meet people with common interests at a local hiking club, religious group, or an adult education class. Participating in new groups or varying your routine can give you the opportunity to meet new people. One patient of mine went to the same church every Sunday for many years. When, for a change of pace, he went to another church, he met the woman who would be his wife. And many meet through Internet sites – which, if the proper precautions are taken, can facilitate connections between people with similar interests.

Friends are often there to help out in a pinch. Sometimes the support is a shoulder to lean on; other times, it is an ear to listen and a heart to care.

## Simplicity

A balancing feat seen on old television shows was spinning plates. The performer would race around spinning one plate on a tall vertical pole, then another, and another.

As a number of plates started spinning, the entertainer would have to go back to the first plates, getting them to spin a little faster. Back and forth he would run, spinning new plates while running back to make sure the old plates were not falling.

The performer looked somewhat entertaining; he looked extremely busy; he may have even looked frantic – he definitely did not look relaxed.

---

**LIFESTYLE TIPS**

## SOCIAL SUPPORT

List what you could do to nurture your current social support system of friends and family:

1. _____

2. _____

3. _____

4. _____

List ways you might expand your social support system (especially if lacking):

1. _____

2. _____

3. _____

4. _____

If you want to be more relaxed, simplicity is key. If you lack basic necessities, more means better. However, in the developed world, many of us would get more happiness from getting rid of items than getting new items. We think that we need the bigger house and more expensive car, so we need to work longer hours, and see our family and friends less. Our balance is off – we're running around trying to keep the plates from falling.

When you're spinning plates, sometimes all you can see is the next plate in danger of falling. People forget to take the time to ask the bigger question: *Is dashing around, spinning plates what I want to do?*

Instead of buying the house or car that you can barely afford, might you be better off giving yourself a little margin? By spending less, you may have to work less, and you will have more time to spend with family and friends.

Decluttering often falls into the category of tough-to-get-started-but-once-I'm-started-satisfying. The key is not to be overwhelmed by a big job, but rather start one drawer at time. If you have half a day to get going, great. If you don't, keep in mind that more often progress is made by setting aside a certain amount of time every day or week that is devoted to decluttering.

Involve the whole family. Teach your children the importance of charity. Will they help by giving away their old, unused toys? If your children are too young to appreciate the logic of giving away their old toys, there is another option. Have them take their old toys to a used toy store. They can go in with a bunch of old toys and get a few dollars to buy a small new toy. If you're still not getting the buy-in and your children are on the young side, put little-used toys away for six months. If your children don't miss them during that period, it might be safe to give them away.

*"Who is rich?*
*He that rejoices in his portion."*
Benjamin Franklin

*"The trouble with the rat race*
*is that even if you win,*
*you're still a rat."*
Lily Tomlin, comedian

## LIFESTYLE TIPS

### SIMPLIFY

List the ways that you could simplify your life:

1. _____

2. _____

3. _____

4. _____

5. _____

## Time Management

Balance is about allocating your time and effort, so having at least a basic understanding of time management skills is paramount. The first skill involves "margin."

Many people attempt to pack their schedules tighter than a rhinoceros in a spandex jumpsuit. It's 9:30 a.m., and you have an 11 a.m. appointment – comfortably, you can fit in those two errands. Yet you try to fit in that one extra chore – the one that ultimately stresses you out and likely makes you late for your appointment.

**Hint One:** If you were flying across the country, would you leave only 10 minutes for a connection between two flights? Not unless you can run a 100-yard dash in five seconds while carrying your luggage in your teeth. You need to leave a little margin in case the first flight is a little late or the gates aren't right next to each other. If you try to continually run your life at maximum capacity, without leaving any room for unexpected occurrences or even room to relax once in a while, you will burn out. In other words, avoid scheduling yourself at 100 percent capacity – leave a little margin.

**Hint Two:** Realize that your inbox will never be empty – be OK with it. The good news is that you don't have to be bored, since, until your last day on Earth, there will always be something to accomplish.

**Hint Three:** Know your priorities. Make a list of the most important things you want to accomplish with your life. Make smaller lists of what you want to accomplish in the next 10 years, five years, one year and next month. Strategize how to make those goals a reality.

**Hint Four:** Have a system – to-do lists, schedules and/ or calendars – some system that works for you. I'm a fan of having my calendar on my smartphone, complete with alerts and alarms, and backed up both on a computer and in the cloud. Of course, that wasn't always my system, because, I was born around the year 12 B.C. – Before Cellular. Back in those days, my system was a calendar and a daily to-do list. If I accomplished a task, it was crossed off the list, and if not, it was transferred to the next day's list. Whatever scheduling system you use, having some system is important. Trust me on this. For example, recently I decided to skip the scheduling system and relied on my memory alone. My son was invited to a party, and I took him there a little early – well ... it was a week early, as it turned out. At least we weren't late.

**Hint Five:** If you can do it fast, do it now. (Unless for some reason you absolutely don't have the time.) If a task can be done in two minutes and it takes 30 seconds to postpone, for the most part, it makes sense to get it over with. I arbitrarily picked out two minutes and 30-second time periods, but perhaps other time periods make sense for you. If you don't have the time to accomplish the task now, put it in your electronic or regular inbox; or, better yet, schedule it.

**Hint Six:** If it's a big project, break it into pieces and schedule time to chip away at it. Tasks such as organizing a house or writing a book likely can't be done in a few hours. However, if you schedule an hour a day to work on a project, you may accomplish more than you thought possible.

**Hint Seven:** Find fun, fast, and relaxing activities. We doctors have a well-deserved reputation for nagging people to avoid harmful habits. Don't smoke! Don't eat foods high in saturated fats! Don't eat too many refined carbohydrates! Don't! Don't! Don't! Although these are all important warnings, perhaps we need to spend more time telling folks what to do – not just what to don't. Do list healthy activities that you enjoy – activities that don't take much time, yet you find relaxing. Petting your dog or cat, gardening, listening to jazz or classical music, going for a walk or a jog, spending time with a loved one. Once you have your list, make sure to scatter these fun relaxing activities throughout your day.

---

### LIFESTYLE TIPS

## LIST FUN, FAST, RELAXING ACTIVITIES

1. _____

2. _____

3. _____

4. _____

5. _____

**LIFESTYLE TIPS**

## LIFE PRIORITY LIST

Take the time to list your life goals and priorities (such as education, family, health, and exercise). Make a "to-do list," and then a daily schedule that includes the most important priorities. You can rank the items A (most important), then B, and finally C (least important). Make sure you include the A priorities in your day, every day. Do not think that marking things with an A ranking means they have to be hard work. Exercise, adequate sleep, and a relaxation exercise are examples of moderate, but advisable, A-priorities.

## Conclusion

Occasionally take the time to reflect on whether your life is in balance. Nurturing a social support network should be a priority, and effective time management skills can help bring a sense of balance back to your life.

# 13

# Technology

On the way back from Zion National Park, my family stayed in a small suite in Las Vegas. Although the suite was small, the bathroom was huge, almost as large as the bedroom and kitchenette combined. The toilet was in a separate room from the sink and shower, and on the counter, next to the sink, was a TV. I thought, "Does there really need to be a television next to a sink? You really can't be away from the TV long enough to wash your face or shave? Really? Besides, when you shave, instead of watching the 'Price is Right,' shouldn't you really be paying attention to your razor-sharp ... well ... razor?"

But who am I kidding? I grew up in a house of multiple televisions. As I went off to college, the constant drone of TV was largely supplanted by incessant stereo music. Silence was rare as a bow-legged snake. Later in my life, after a decades-long remission from a TV addiction, the smartphone revolution occurred.

It's bad enough to check your phone while out and about, but – more than once – I've checked my smartphone while standing up to urinate. One day, after relieving myself, I dropped my cell phone in the toilet. I wondered, "How did that happen?" I usually wasn't clumsy enough to let a phone slide right through my hands and it didn't seem like I had lost my grip, but I could find no other logical explanation for the wet phone. I made a mental note: "Be more careful next time." I dried my phone and miraculously, it worked. Next time my bladder called, I stood up, unzipped, started the stream, checked my email on the phone, and, when I finished, very, very carefully placed the phone in my front shirt pocket. Gravity's acceleration rate of 32 feet per second squared went into effect as my phone fell through a hole at the bottom of the pocket, down, down, down, with a resounding kerplunk. Mystery solved! Had I not been operating on complete automatic pilot, I would have discovered the defective pocket the first go around and been spared the need to replace the phone, now soaked beyond resuscitation.

There are certainly many ways we greatly benefit from digital technology; we have access to an incredible wealth of knowledge, the ability to almost instantaneously communicate across the globe, and stupid cat videos. What technology has failed to provide is the common sense to know when to turn it off. In fact, technology, driven by advertising revenue and crafty marketing specialists, has a vested interested in keeping our eyes glued to screens both large and small.

Having some time when one is not immersed in technology can pay off in relaxation gold. How much technology-free time (TFT) might we need? If nothing else, let's start by at least taking a break long enough to take a whiz. Generally speaking, relieving a full bladder feels good – you might as well enjoy it.

People check their phones non-stop: in the middle of an "intimate" dinner – checking email; on a nature hike – posting a pic on Facebook; in bed with your spouse –

Twittering or texting away. And then there is the truly dangerous: using a phone while driving, a habit that has cost many lives. Thus, the importance of TFT ranges from creating more enjoyment in life, to being more effective in work, to even saving lives.

Some may choose to set aside one whole day a week, or the Sabbath, to disconnect from technology. Alternatively, you might set aside a small amount of time every day to be free of the digital stream. Pick out some activities that should have less technology and more mindfulness. Possibilities include: at the dinner table, other meals, times of intimate communication or sex or perhaps when you first wake up or right before you go to sleep.

In general, when you really want to accomplish a task, having a tech-free period may make a lot of sense. Although society values multitasking, multitasking is largely an illusion. Our brains work most effectively by fully focusing on one task. When someone talks on the phone, while watching TV and answering an email, he may seem to be doing all of those things at once, but what he is really doing is very quickly shifting his attention from one task, to another, and back again. Phone, TV, email, TV, phone, TV, email, and on and on. The problem is that every time we shift our attention, we must take a moment to reorient – "Where was I again?" Thus, when people attempt to multitask, they tend to be less, not more, efficient.

Digital devices can also affect personal relationships. We now have wonderful ways to connect to people electronically. However, there is something special and unique about a face-to-face chat, and nothing says

"I care" like giving your full and complete attention to your friend.

If you are sitting on hold on a telephone for 10 minutes, sure, get some reading done. However, one time I called someone, and while the phone was ringing, I started at some other task and forgot whom I called. With the speed of snail, I queried, "Hellooo, maaay I pleeeaaasse speee-aaak wiiiiith ...," followed by an abrupt and barely intel-ligible, "Sorry, I'll have to call back later." Can you say "embarrassing"? How about "inefficient"? Or "waste of time"? This was the extreme.

Usually, devoting 20 to 30 fully focused minutes to one task will increase your work efficacy. If you are an ambulance driver, you really need to answer the emer-gency call on the double. However, unless you are a TMZ reporter, checking that celebrity tweet is really not an emergency – keep working. After a 20 to 30 minute burst of work, a little change of focus may be in order.

Although, I'm using the term "technology-free time," perhaps it would better to use the term "reality-full time." Instead of being perpetually lost in the virtual world, reserve time to mindfully immerse yourself in the "real world."

---

**Practice**

# TFT

Brainstorm to find some possible technology-free times:

1. _____

2. _____

3. _____

4. _____

5. _____

---

## Television

In 2003, our family owned a humongous, whale-size TV, left over from my bachelor days. It was 37 times the bulk and weight of my then-2-year-old twin boys, twins known for their legendary destructive teamwork, a partnership that had enabled them to destroy an entire closet, including the closet's high shelves. They did so by scaling dizzying heights that no lone child could even dream of reaching. The potential danger posed by the enormous TV was obvious. It had to go. (We first heard of the danger of big televisions falling and injuring young children on the television. An appliance was asking for its own removal, kind of like a toaster printing a letter of resignation on a piece of bread.)

When we gave away the whale-size TV, there was no back-up. The plan was to get one of those newfangled flat-screen TVs, until we learned at that time they came with a four-grand price tag. "Hmm, what to do? What to do?" As we mulled that question, time passed, and there was one thing we didn't miss: TV.

In giving up TV, we didn't totally go back to the Stone Age; we still had a dishwasher, washing machine, and computer. Not infrequently, we'd hook up a digital projector to the computer and enjoy movies and other shows. The fact that it took more than a push of a button to access our video entertainment meant we avoided the temptation to have the tube on non-stop or to waste time with any old, low-quality audio-visual dreck.

Our solution to the TV issue may not be the best one for all families. However, since frequent TV-watchers are fatter and more likely to develop serious health issues including diabetes, coming up with some solution or plan is important. Your solution may be a modest one, such as getting the TV out of the bedroom, unless you find that the 11 o'clock news really spices up your romantic life. Nothing like a weather report to get you all hot and bothered.

Other topics on the evening news will truly just get you plain bothered. It makes sense to not only be careful about how you feed your body, but also be aware of how you feed your mind. I've seen many people who add considerably to their stress level with their insatiable appetite for violent shows, both dramas and the daily news. These shows keep the fear factor turned up as high as possible with the hope you will stay tuned. Thus, you are not only disturbed, but your view of life is distorted into a scarier and more pessimistic outlook. Unless you are unusually sensitive, it's not necessary to avoid all news and scary movies. Just be aware of how much you partake, and that shows aim to emphasize and inflate the drama and suspense.

If you are used to non-stop TV in the background, breaks from it may initially feel odd. But, if not immediately, then after a time, you'll begin to notice and enjoy wonderful sounds, sights, tastes, and fragrances that emerge when your consciousness is not otherwise engaged.

If there's a TV show you love to watch, by all means, enjoy. Just be wise about what you watch and how much you watch. There are often more relaxing ways to spend your time than surfing through 500 channels without reward, only to do it again and again.

## Back it Up

Life has changed. For the most part, closets crammed with leather-bound books full of plastic-encased photos have gone the way of the rotary phone. Now, treasured photos, music collections, and important family and work records all live on the computer. And that computer won't work forever. Indeed, your hard drive will crash, the thumb drive will fall off your keychain, and/or your laptop will be stolen.

Drive a car long enough and it will break down; use a computer long enough and ditto. On the plus side, you can easily prevent the stress of such a meltdown.

## BACK UP YOUR DATA

There are many ways to back up your data, and in the time it takes to write this paragraph, even better ways will have been created. Each way has its advantages and disadvantages, and therefore, ideally, it's best to pick more than one way to back up your information. Just a few of the currently available choices include:

1. Using an external hard drive. This is relatively inexpensive and both backup and restoration can be done quickly.

2. Using a service that does backup over the Internet. On the downside, when the backup occurs, your computer may be a little slower. On the upside, the backup is automatic so you don't have to worry about forgetting. Also, it is off site, so even if you have a robbery or fire, your information is safe.

3. Currently, many services such as Google will give you a certain amount of backup space for free. If you save your data to your "Google Drive," a copy will be automatically saved off site and available to access from computers away from home.

## Virtual Comparisons

On occasion, surely even cavemen were jealous. After all, Zock had such a cool spear, and did you see how talented his kid was at cave painting? Jump ahead a million years, and it's not just our neighbor we might envy, but we can now be jealous of millions of people – from an old elementary school acquaintance to a celebrity halfway around the world.

The Internet, TV and smartphones have revolutionized the art of envy. We can now compare our lives with countless others, whose lives, distorted by our media, seem so much better than ours. We compare our bodies to pictures of models, whose job it is to stay in shape, dressed by professional designers, face-painted by professional makeup artists, and whose pictures are then Photoshopped to extremes of "perfection," unattainable by any normal human.

On social networking sites, people compare their lives with those of friends and old classmates, who largely report only the interesting and usually good news. We hear all about our old classmate's wonderful week of vacation, and little about the other 51 weeks of doing things like folding the laundry.

And the biggest distortion of all – that happiness comes from wealth and fame. Although we might assert, "Money doesn't buy happiness," that doesn't stop us from coveting a costly car, magnificent mansion, or decadent diamond doodad. Many believe that the way to happiness is money and sex, but at least one study showed that it wasn't billionaire playboys who best lit up their pleasure centers. Functional MRI and EEG studies with monks – who had few worldly possessions and no sex whatsoever – showed the highest-ever measured activity of the left prefrontal cortex, currently the prime objective indicator for happiness.

One reason celebrity "news" is so popular is that it fuels people's imagination of living a luxurious lifestyle. Another reason is the hunger to watch the rich and famous fail, temporarily shattering the happiness-for-a-price illusion.

Much of this illusion is no accident. Once people have their basic food and shelter needs met, having more stuff brings just a transient increase in happiness. However, the level soon returns to the baseline. Advertisers want you to spend, so they need to convince you that you can't live without the latest thingamajig, or at least that your life would be immeasurably better with it. To get as much of your money as they can, they might offer a baseline product and then convince you how much happier you would be with each upgrade. As the rock group Styx sang about years ago, this the "Grand Illusion."

Add the grass-is-greener-on-the-other-side distortion to the greener-grass-brings-happiness fallacy and you get the great green-eyed monster of envy. Trying to beat out, or match everyone on the Internet and TV works about as well for achieving happiness as an all-you-can-eat doughnut-and-ice-cream diet works for trimming your waistline.

What does work? Mindfulness and gratitude of just this moment – available here and now, free of charge.

A recent study suggested that people who spent more time on Facebook tended to be sadder. However, there is a way to turn that around and instead feel more joyous and compassionate after a session on social media.

## IN CONTRAST TO COMPARING
## – BE MINDFUL

If you start being bummed or stressed that others seem to have more than you, remember that true happiness comes from being mindful of this moment – focus on the enjoyment of this breath or this bite of food, etc. Remind yourself of all your blessings. It's funny how people notice those who have more than they do, while they fail to notice the many who lack the basic necessities of food and shelter. List your blessings: food, shelter, friends, family, your ability to see and hear, and on, and on.

Practice

## SOCIAL MEDIA AS AN EXERCISE
## IN COMPASSION

As you get updates on your social network, use that time to strengthen your ability to be compassionate and to have joy in others' accomplishments. If you read sad news, think to yourself, "May his suffering decrease." Say it to yourself as earnestly and with as much feeling as possible. Each time something good happens, in the same way think: "May your good fortune continue; may your happiness continue and grow."

When you do this, you will end the session at social media happier, more compassionate, and more relaxed.

## Summary

When you are a slave to technology, you might yearn for simpler times. However, in reality, few of us would really want to do without the tech conveniences we've become accustomed to. The novelty of the good old prehistoric days would probably wear off as quickly as you can say, "Cappuccino, please." Developing the discipline to be a master of technology, instead of a slave to technology, will allow you to have the best of modern times, while still treasuring life's simple moments.

# 14

# Less Stress Nutrition

*"I went on a diet. Had to go on two diets at the same time 'cause one wasn't giving me enough food."*
Barry Mater

Many women, sooner or later, ask the question, "Does this dress make me look fat," and all men over 25 have learned that there is only one correct response to this question – quickly and convincingly saying, "No, honey, you look great!" Although I've learned the hard way that you may want to hesitate just long enough to actually look at the woman before replying. My son was much younger than 25 when his not-overweight-at-all mother asked: "Does this dress make me look fat?" As I was applying my hesitate-just-long-enough-to-look technique, my son responded: "Not as fat as Dad." I had to finally admit that my abdomen was appearing somewhat less like a six-pack, and somewhat more like a full keg. If I didn't get things under control soon, I knew that my next weigh-in would need to be on a Richter scale.

Indeed, as I was rounding half a century, my own belly was getting significantly rounder. I also had been suffering from the middle-age guy's version of an altered body image perception. The teenage girl's version deservingly gets lots of press: typically, the teen is carbon-nanotube thin, and she thinks she's obese. The typical middle-age guy (MAG) problem is the reverse: We think we're lean and athletic – as we sport our Santa-size waists.

Now, we don't come down too hard on us MAGs. Not only do we have to contend with possible faults in our genes, we also have faults in our jeans. Just as the fashion industry conspires against girls in their teens, the jeans companies conspire against MAGs. How else can you explain a guy with a 38-inch waist being able to fit into 34-inch jeans? We can delude ourselves at the mirror by sucking our in guts so far that our eyes pop out. Thus, not only does our waist look slightly less protuberant, but vision is obscured by our eyes being slightly out of socket. A candid photo might shock us into reality, but we're convinced that the camera angle must have been off, and I seem to remember something in physics class about "refraction" causing optical illusions. After all, my jeans can't lie; can they?

A rough guideline to see if you need to lose weight entails measuring your waist, not – I said NOT – just going by the label on your jeans, but actually measuring your waist size. If your waist circumference is more than half your height (meaning a ratio of over 0.5), losing some weight may be a way to gain better health. Just because you don't feel a bunch of jiggly blubber on the outside doesn't mean things are fine on the inside. In fact, a layer of fat surrounding your internal organs, but inside your abdominal wall muscles, is far more dangerous than a layer of cellulite on your thighs.

If your waist size is a lot more than half your height, don't panic. If you are markedly overweight, even losing 10 pounds can decrease your blood pressure and likely cut your risk of stroke. In the same vein, if your waist circumference-to-height ratio is 0.8, getting it down to 0.75 will improve your health and be an excellent beginning to your ultimate goal.

Author Michael Pollan stated the simplest rules for nutrition: "Eat food, not too much, and mostly plants." (And by "food," Michael Pollan means the type of real food your great-grandmother would recognize – the food on the outer edge of the grocery store instead of the highly processed food-like stuff-with-ingredients-you-can't-pronounce in the middle of the store.) And add one more rule: Pay attention when you're eating so you can enjoy your food. These rules apply whether you need to lose weight or not.

Some of the information in the rest of this chapter is general nutrition advice. Since two-thirds of the U.S. population is either overweight or obese, and since weight-loss is a stressful issue for many, I have also included advice more geared for people who want to lose weight. For those who want more nutrition information, keep reading.

## Mindful Eating

Think of the first time you tried wine – not the sweet stuff, but a regular merlot or chardonnay. When I was young, my initial reaction was not yum, but yuck! It is not until later that people typically develop a taste for wine. Wine connoisseurs carefully and slowly appreciate each sip of wine. They enjoy the appearance of the wine. They dwell on its bouquet and they savor one small sip. And, indeed, that is why they enjoy the wine. The way one drinks the wine has as much or more to do with the enjoyment than does the label on the bottle. And the same goes for the enjoyment of food – how one eats is at least as important as what one eats.

Most often, people don't savor each bite of food like they would taste a fine wine. Much of the time, people hardly taste their food at all. If you find a good part of the potato chip bag empty and have crumbs on your mouth, but you didn't taste one bite, you've been cruising on automatic pilot. Although it may be against the law to drive while distracted, you won't get arrested for eating while distracted. However, it can certainly decrease your enjoyment of food while adding to your waistline.

Don't give yourself a hard time. Have reasonable expectations – just as you are frequently not mindful of your breathing, you won't always be mindful of your eating. The first step to mindful eating is to realize when you are rushing around like the Not-Fast-Enough-Food Guy in Chapter 11. Recognize the feeling of urgency in your eating. Once you've realize that you're being all NFEFG, you're most of the way there. Feel the breath in your abdomen, and perhaps relax a muscle group with your exhalation. Then, really taste your food. Appreciate the appearance of the food. Enjoy the aroma. Luxuriate in the taste and texture of just this bite. Put your fork down between bites, and slow down. If it's a special treat, you might even close your eyes to fully tune into your senses of smell and taste.

When it comes to enjoying a meal, how we eat is at least as important as what we eat. Eating is one of our great sensual pleasures. If we eat a ton of calories without even noticing, what hope have we got to lose weight?

With my knowledge of mindful eating and nutrition, I decided to try just a couple of rules to help me lose weight:

1. **Eat real, nutritious food** – lay off of candy, cakes, etc.

2. **Eat mindfully** – no eating standing up. No eating while reading, while on the computer, or while watching television. As much as possible I tried to pay attention to and enjoy each bite.

For me, (and many others) those two simple rules weren't quite enough, but the weight did indeed come off with a bit of work and one additional rule: **Keep track.**

If one wants to lose weight, it makes sense to keep track of calorie intake and expenditure. Research shows that when people keep track of their food intake they can double their weight loss. Enter technology – several smartphone apps make watching your calories simple. Type in a few letters or scan a package bar code, and voila! Apps such as, "MyFitnessPal.com" or "Lose It!" give you enough information to lose weight. And keeping track of what you eat does indeed make you more mindful of what you eat. Instead of eating a bag of pistachios in front of the TV, you note that 10 nuts have 40 calories, count out perhaps 20 nuts and put the bag away before eating. Thereby, you become more mindful not only of what you eat, but also of how much you eat.

Keeping track of what you eat is also a learning experience. Do I really want to eat that rich dip, or is the 10-calorie-a-serving salsa a wiser (and just as tasty) choice? One guy I know lost about a pound a week just by substituting some mustard instead of his usual glob of mayonnaise on his daily sandwich, and by trading salads slathered with high-calorie dressing in for salads with a little low-cal dressing.

The phone app would lead me to choose having one slice of pizza with a really big salad. Prior to this, pizzas would fear me. Their little pepperoni knees would tremble, for I would devour half a large pizza before you could say "mozzarella."

By inputting information in real time (or close to it), even someone with a Ph.D. in nutrition is bound to learn. A good friend of mine would get her favorite salad at a popular restaurant chain on a weekly basis. Her frustration with weight loss led her to start using a calorie tracking app when lo and behold ... that salad ... for we were taught salads are for dieters ... that salad ... ready for it ... had 1300 calories. This salad did not put her on the track to trim, but was rather the path to plump. And she learned that just because a meal has the word "salad" in it doesn't mean it's healthy. In this case, it was almost her whole day's calorie budget on one plate.

At first, journaling either in a notebook or with the help of smartphone app may seem cumbersome. However, when you make it a habit, keeping track can be relatively seamless. Additionally, several of the smartphone apps show you how exercise fits into the weight loss regime. Exercise more, and you can eat more and still make your goal.

You will be more successful if you can make keeping track of your calories into a game. The smartphone apps, with their ease of use and various features, can help encourage this game mentality. When discussing someone's diet, often I hear, "I know what to do; I just don't do it." Keeping track of calories and making sport of it may provide the extra motivation you need.

Just the thought of keeping track of your food intake may provide insight. Not infrequently, I've had patients claim to have a stellar diet, no clue how they could not lose weight, until I asked them to keep track of their diet, and then: "Well I do munch on trail mix throughout my day at work," or "I do have a soda, or two, in the afternoon." Aha. Mystery solved.

Eating mindfully is, in general, slower than speed eating in front of the computer. If you doubled the pace of your eating, you might think you would finish your meal twice as quickly. That would be the case if you ate the same amount of food. However, when people eat more quickly, they tend to eat more. It takes some time (often quoted as about 20 minutes) for the brain to register feeling full. If you double your eating speed but cram in twice the amount of food, really no time is saved. Although the fast, mindless eating didn't cut your meal time in half, it will double your waistline and triple your heartburn.

Remembering to eat slower has historically been a problem for me. I try a few principles, and recommend them to you:

1. Before eating, try taking a couple of mindful diaphragmatic breaths and notice if you are hungry. If not, the plan is to postpone eating, if possible. People eat out of habit or to deal with stress, sadness, or other emotions.

2. Slow your meal down a bit – get in the habit of putting down your fork between bites and

taking one or two deep diaphragmatic breaths after every several bites. Occasionally, evaluate your level of hunger. Some people end their meal when they are "full," but by that they mean "stuffed." The sign that you are full should not be that you can't possibly force another bite into your mouth. Rather, I advise people to stop eating as soon as the hunger sensation begins to subside. Put the food away, or get up from the table to discourage mindless nibbling. Consider taking a break from the table, when you are not quite full, and savor a warm cup of tea. This style of eating encourages the healthy routine of eating small, frequent meals.

3. Keeping track of your meals with a journal or with a smartphone app will also help you slow down.

## Veggies

With all that being said, there are times when my schedule seems too hectic to eat slowly and mindfully with focused attention. Perhaps I'm busy at work, hungry, but just don't have the time for a relaxed meal. And that is why God made vegetables. If you insist on some mindless quick eating as you work on the computer, don't quickly consume chocolates. You're not tasting the food anyway, so what's the point? Keep something like carrots, snap peas, celery or baby tomatoes around. If you aren't taking the time to really appreciate food, for broccoli's sake, don't eat calorie-dense goodies. Save the fudge for when you can close your eyes, whiff the aroma, and feel the texture and taste of each little mini bite.

I try to keep some raw veggies by my desk. It's easier to resist eating the whole bag of chips when I'm not famished. Having my gut at least partly satiated with nutritious food helps me avoid DDDD – Distracted Dorito Devouring Disorder. If someone brings a special high-calorie treat into the office, instead quickly consuming three slices of pie, I close my eyes and luxuriate in the taste of a quarter-slice.

Get at least five fist-size servings of vegetables into your diet. Vegetables tend to be low in calories and high in nutrients and fiber. Science has made great strides in isolating various nutrients and putting them into supplements. However, it would be arrogant to think that we've found all the important nutrients contained in various vegetables. There are certain micro nutrients that just aren't available in a supplement. Which ones? Primarily the ones we haven't yet discovered. In summary, if you just can't muster getting the veggies in, a vitamin/mineral supplement might be a good idea. However, it's not a substitute for the real food.

Pick a variety of vegetables. And no – carrot cake is not considered a vegetable. Also, most of our diets contain plenty of potatoes and corn, so focus more on other veggies. In fact, the documentary "King Corn" starts with a hair analysis of two typical men. Over 50 percent of the carbon in their bodies came from corn. How is that possible? They didn't eat 12 ears of corn on the cob daily. They didn't, but most of the meat they ate came from corn-fed animals. And, largely because of corn subsidies, high fructose corn syrup seems to sweeten a wide gamut of food products. So, in essence, we are composed largely of corn – which gives a whole new meaning for being corny.

(While the last sentence relies on the old standard meaning of being corny.) So, for the most part, let's consider corn and potatoes starch. And let's try to increase the intake of other vegetables.

## Carbs

In general, it's best to limit your intake of starches or high-carbohydrate foods, such as bread, pasta or rice. When you do eat grains, instead of refined carbs (such as sugary foods, white bread, white rice or white pasta), choose the whole grain products. The refined carbs result in a high peak blood sugar, which in turn causes a higher blood insulin response. The blood sugar drops and your body often responds by releasing extra stress hormones to increase the blood sugar.

## Don't Skip

These stress hormones also respond to other drops of blood sugar, which is one of the reasons why skipping breakfast, or another meal for that matter, will make people into cranksters.

Perhaps you think that a little irritability is worth some weight loss. Think again, Mr. Got-morning-breath-at-noon! Research by epidemiologist Mark Pereira Ph.D. (sponsored by the American Heart Association) showed that people who regularly ate breakfast had a much lower incidence of obesity than people who did not regularly eat breakfast. People who ate breakfast regularly also had a lower risk of prediabetes. If there is absolutely no time for a meal, a meal substitute (such as a protein drink or bar) is better than skipping breakfast completely.

## Protein

Part of a balanced diet includes adequate protein – not a problem for most burger-eating folks in the U.S. Lean meats, fish and chicken are all reasonable sources of protein. Beans, nuts, and dairy also provide protein, giving vegetarians good options. Decreasing the amount of protein you get from meat has some additional bonuses:

1. Non-meat sources of protein lack the high saturated fat content present in fatty meats.

2. Growing plants consumes many times less natural resources than does the raising of animals for meat. According to some sources, it takes approximately 2,000 gallons of water to produce each pound of meat.

3. Methane is at least 25 times more potent in causing global warming than is carbon dioxide, which would be just another boring fact if it weren't for one thing – cows produce a lot of methane. In fact, the raising of livestock produces more greenhouse gas (measured in carbon dioxide equivalents) than does all transportation combined.

## Fluids

And that brings us to hydration: If you drink a gallon of eggnog a day there will be some benefit ... to the eggnog salesman. You, on the other hand, will need to save up for your cardiac bypass surgery. So, I guess the heart surgeon might benefit as well.

Fluids are great for quenching your thirst, however drinks don't tend to satisfy your appetite like solid food.

You can quench your thirst with no calories – when you're parched, it's hard to beat an ice cold glass of water; when you want to relax on a cold morning, a warm cup of tea can be most excellent. If you don't want to gain weight, it makes sense to get most of your hydration from calorie-free or low-calorie drinks.

Perhaps you say, "Wait ... juice is healthy. It's not like soda." Think again. Drink 16 ounces of apple juice and you'll get several apples worth of sugar and about 250 calories. The apple juice may quench your thirst, but will do virtually nothing to fill you up. Compare that to eating a medium apple that contains about 80 calories and also contains a bunch of healthy fiber that can satisfy your appetite. Unless you are desperately trying to gain weight, the better choice is really a no-brainer.

## Obstacles

Anticipate potential problems ahead of time and have strategies to overcome them. For instance, if people tend to bring in doughnuts to work, make sure you bring in some healthly snacks.

When you "fall off the wagon," be easy on yourself and don't give yourself too much of a hard time. Research shows that piling on the guilt just increases the risk that you'll pile on the pounds. So forgive your failings, see what you can learn from your errors, and start fresh.

## Avoiding Excess Alcohol, Caffeine, or Drugs

*Stan was about 30 years old and was suffering*
*from what appeared to be severe panic attacks.*
*Before prescribing the medications typically used*
*for panic attacks, I asked him how much coffee he*

*drank. "Three a day" was his answer. I told him*
*that three cups of coffee per day could certainly in-*
*crease a person's anxiety level. Then Stan clarified*
*his response: It was three pots of coffee a day.*

It's no mystery that too much caffeine can put the edge in edgy. And what is too much? No easy answer to that. People have varying sensitivities to caffeine. Even a serving or two a day can cause problems for some people. One problem is that people are often confused as to what constitutes a serving.

Does anyone really need to drink a 64-ounce soda with more than five times the caffeine and sugar of a standard 12-ounce soda? Coffee sizes are also problematic. My fifth-grade math teacher said that a cup is 8 fluid ounces and my Mr. Coffee pot tells me a cup is 6 ounces. Even using the larger of those two standards, a typical coffee shop sizes contain 1 1/2 cups, 2 cups, and 2 1/2 cups of coffee. In other words, two large cups of coffee is really 5 cups of coffee – and according to a Mr. Coffee pot, it's almost 7 cups of coffee.

I'm not suggesting that everyone abstain from caffeine; in fact, a 2013 study suggested that a cup of coffee a day, or 4 cups of green tea, might offer protection from stroke. What I am suggesting is that you be aware of what constitutes a cup, and that you have some awareness of your individual sensitivity to caffeine.

The discussion of measurement is relevant to alcohol as well. "Frank, how much beer do you drink?" Frank responds, "Not much." On clarification, Frank's "not much" equals a case of beer a day. And why shouldn't he think a case of beer is not much? After all, most of his buddies drink that much or more. The norms of alcohol intake among different groups of people vary widely. Despite varying norms, excessive alcohol can have adverse effects on both the body and the mind.

A healthy intake of alcohol is zero to two drinks per day. And a drink does not mean a six-pack of beer, bottle of wine or pint of vodka. A drink is 12 ounces of beer, a 5-ounce glass of wine, or 1.5 ounces of hard alcohol. As people age, the tolerance for alcohol decreases, so for a 70-year-old a limit of one drink per day makes sense. For people with certain medical conditions, like liver disease, abstaining from alcohol altogether is probably the best choice.

Many heavy drinkers are surrounded by friends who also drink heavily, and they may have difficulty recognizing that they have a problem with alcohol. Recovery from alcohol addiction often requires that people find new social support groups. Alcoholics Anonymous is one group that serves this function well.

Several so-called recreational drugs can also cause increased anxiety. Cocaine and amphetamines can cause severe anxiety and panic. Even a single use of these drugs can cause a heart attack or seizure. Illegal drugs are not the only drugs that make people anxious. Certain decongestants, asthma medications, antidepressants, and appetite suppressants can cause excessive anxiety in susceptible individuals. If you suspect this type of problem with a prescribed medication, discuss the issue with your doctor before discontinuing it.

## Body Image

Earlier in the chapter, I joked about us middle age guys looking in the mirror and not seeing our bellies. On the other hand, there are folks at a healthy weight, but because of a desire to be skinnier, they starve themselves and/or hate themselves.

If you have questions about your healthy weight, check in with your health care provider. BMI calculations and body fat measurements, although imperfect, can help guide that determination. As mentioned earlier, a relatively easy guideline to find a healthy weight is by checking that your waist circumference is approximately half of your height. Obsessing about looking just like a pencil-thin model can cause both physical and emotional problems. It's much cheaper to just buy some Photoshop software – after all, that's what they do.

> **Optional Audio Exercise:** eating meditation available at www.RelaxationOnTheRun.com

## Less Stress Diet Summary

1. When possible, eat slowly and mindfully.

2. Eat lots of veggies. If you don't have time to eat mindfully, eat veggies.

3. If you want to lose weight, track your eating and consider a smartphone app to help with this. Turn making your calorie goals into a game.

4. Recognize the tendency to quickly eat like NFEFG, and then take some mindful breaths.

5. Avoid skipping meals.

6. Make most of your fluid intake or calorie-free or at least low-calorie (such as water or herbal tea.)

7. Avoid excessive alcohol or caffeine.

8. Depending on your tendencies, it may be best to buy little or none in the way of high-calorie treats for home. Why make it too easy to go off track?

9. If your nutrition plan goes awry, don't be a hater. Give yourself some slack, be kind to yourself, learn from any mistakes and restart a little wiser.

10. Also, when you run into a problem with your diet, reread this chapter, or if you are too busy for that at least read the summary again. Resolve to follow the guidelines for a day, or even a meal, and give yourself credit for doing so. Regain that momentum.

# 15

# Less Stress Exercise

The fight-or-flight response, as its name implies, evolved as a way to prepare us for physical exertion. And after physical exertion, the adrenaline levels decreases and we feel more relaxed. Yet, for most of us, today's world involves much more sitting than running. We've covered a variety of ways to relax, but we should not forget that physical exercise remains an important way to reduce stress.

Exercise can improve health, well-being, longevity, and happiness. As far as antidepressants go, exercise is as natural as it gets.

In this chapter we will explore the basic components of a good exercise program and a variety of exercise options. How can you make exercise more enjoyable? How, with a busy schedule, can you find the time to exercise? There are many forms of exercise; if you chose to run/jog, how can you do it and decrease risk of injury?

And let's start with: "How much should you exercise?" And the good news is, it doesn't have to be that much. A 2015 study looked into the optimal amount of jogging needed to maximize longevity. It comes as no surprise that sedentary people do not live as long as people who exercise. It also should not be a surprise that you can overdo it, and by exercising too much, you can actually risk your health. According to the aforementioned study, the peak exercise benefit occurred when study participants jogged at a slow to moderate pace for 1 to 2.4 hours per week with the optimal frequency of jogging being two to three times per week.

There were some faults with the above study, and given the number of people in each group we can be more confident saying jogging at least an hour a week is helpful and less confident that people should not jog more than 2.4 hours a week. The big takeaway here is that just a little exercise can drastically improve your health and longevity. Most folks can find the time to put in 20 minutes of exercise three days a week.

There are three components to a healthy exercise program:

1. Aerobic exercise.

2. Keeping your body limber with stretching
   (and consider balance exercises).

3. Building strength.

This chapter does not include extensive instruction in all forms of exercise – not even close. Rather, it has a few pearls about exercise, hopefully some of which will be useful to you.

## Aerobic Exercise

If you enjoy exercising, you're more likely to do it. If you don't swim like a fish or a run like a gazelle, or if rowing doesn't float your boat, there's still something for you. For at least 20 minutes three days a week, find a way to exercise – hiking, dancing, tennis, taking the baby jogger out ... find something you enjoy.

For those who like to run/jog, recommendations have changed since I was in high school cross country. Back then, with each stride we were advised to land on our heel and roll forward. And my high school knees did fine with such a stride; however, my middle-age knees – not so much. Landing on the heels is a good way to maximize the impact forces going up your knees, hips and lower back. Research has shown that using a "mid-foot strike" will decrease injury.

Assume a good standing posture – upright with shoulders back. Then lean your whole body forward and naturally let one of your legs come forward in your stride. The mid-foot should contact the ground with the knee slightly bent. In that way, the whole foot and the leg become a shock absorber.

Another trend in exercise is wearable technology. Devices can range from a simple pedometer to the more complex that collects much more data, including number of stairs climbed, heart rate, and GPS location. A popular way to encourage people to be more active is to ask them to take a minimum number of steps – a common goal being 10,000 steps a day. For some, just getting to 5,000 steps a day would be a worthy goal. These wearable tech devices have the added advantage of encouraging reframing. Have to park far away? That's not a bummer; it's a great chance to increase your steps for that day.

## Stretching

I never felt competitive with my flexibility – namely because I'd lose a stretching contest with a two-inch-thick iron rod.

I have realized that stretching is important. Some degree of flexibility helps prevent injury. The old recommendation of stretching before a workout is ... well ... old. You don't want to stretch cold muscles. The simplest way around this is just stretch at the end of your aerobic exercise. At least a short bit of aerobic exercise is recommended to warm up your muscles prior to stretching.

Mindful stretching, AKA yoga, has been practiced for thousands of years. This trend is a keeper, and rightly so. What are the advantages of bringing mindfulness to stretching?

- By stretching mindfully, you're bound to be more careful and less likely to tear your groin muscles from jumping into a split.

- By practicing mindfulness in another setting besides sitting, it increases your ability to bring mindfulness to your daily life.

- Mindfulness can turn a stretching into a relaxation break.

- By learning to mindfully deal with the mild discomfort of a stretch, one can use the practice skills to deal with other discomforts through the day.

As you practice mindful stretching, patiently bring your attention back to your breath and/or the sensations of your body. Notice if your body tenses when your stretch. Does your jaw or neck tighten as you stretch your leg? If so, allow those muscles to relax. Perhaps as you stretch your hamstrings, notice your abdomen as you breathe in and allow your hamstrings to further relax each time you exhale. At times, become aware of your whole body as you stretch.

Work on keeping your flexibility symmetric. Speaking from personal experience: one tight left hamstring + one tight right quadriceps = one sore low back. So if you notice one side tighter than the other, spend a bit more time stretching the tighter side.

And it doesn't take a ton of time. Yes; there are some who practice 90 minutes of yoga a day. If you can do that, great. If not, I bet you can spare five minutes three days a week.

For each exercise, 20 to 30 seconds per side can help keep you a bit more limber. And, as mentioned, if one side is a little tighter, give that side an extra turn. And, finally, by all means, stretch gently, slowly and mindfully. And if you start getting any sharp or severe pain, stop right away.

There are multiple ways to stretch a muscle group; Here are a few examples:

The first stretch is my favorite and my name for it will give you a hint why I like it so much – "The Lazy Hamstring Stretch." After some aerobic exercise to warm up your muscles, lie down on your back next to a doorway. One leg extends out the doorway and the other goes up the wall adjacent to the door frame. Relax that way for 20 or 30 seconds and switch legs. (Be aware of what's going on at the other side of the door. Although someone tripping over your leg may be funny in a slapstick way, if that person breaks a hip, it's not quite as funny.)

Next is the quadriceps stretch: Face the front of a chair or sofa and place your hands on it for stability. Bend your left knee, and put the front of the right knee on the floor. Extend your right leg back and bend your left knee further – you should feel the stretch on the right hamstring. Then switch sides.

To stretch your calf muscles, put both hands against a wall or a desk, and put your right leg further back. Keep your right foot flat on the floor as you extend your right leg back far enough until you feel the stretch. The calf stretch should be done with back leg straight and then again with a slight bend of the back knee. Then switch sides.

The piriformis stretch I enjoy is another that lets me lie on my back. Bend your left leg and initially keep the left foot on the ground. Cross your right ankle over your left knee. Lock your hands behind your left thigh and gently pull. Your left foot may raise off the ground. Then switch sides.

In addition to stretching, balance exercises can be beneficial. Tai Chi, a practice including mindful movement and balance, is very helpful for a variety of problems including fall prevention.

## Strength Training

You don't need biceps the size of watermelons. But do you really want to have to beg others to open that pickle jar for you? Strength training can help keep both your bones and muscles strong. Forgo this type of exercise and you may be on the road to osteoporosis (weak bones) and the lesser-known sarcopenia (loss of muscle mass and strength).

Notice that I said "a little strength training." Options include 15 to 20 minutes on some resistance machines at a health club a couple times a week, or just a regimen at home with push-ups, pull-ups and some core exercises. Although the scope of this chapter does not allow for much depth, let me include just a few hints:

1. Technique is vital. When I was in my mid-20s, I could bench press 180 percent of my body weight. Did that make me more awesome? Not "more awesome," but rather it made me "more onic" − aka moronic. My form was awful. I'd bounce the barbell off my chest to be able to somehow manage one repetition. Poor form is a one-way ticket to injury. In other words, leave your ego at the door. Instead of lifting the maximum weight, do the exercises with slow, controlled, mindful movements. Get instruction from someone who knows what to do and have have him or her observe that you are doing the exercises correctly. In general, most exercises are done for 10 to 20 repetitions. Some muscle soreness and fatigue can be normal, but sharp pain is not. Any pain that is severe or sharp means stop. Even if an exercise is done with correct form, if it is causing severe pain it is likely not the exercise for you. Each person's body is different, so an exercise that is perfect for Jim may be perfectly awful for John.

2. If you're busy, make use of your downtime. Typically, people do multiple sets of a given exercise, and each set consists of several reps or repetitions. In between sets, people will rest the involved muscle group. As you rest one muscle

group, you can exercise another. You could alternate an arm exercise with a leg or abdominal exercise. Alternatively, you could do a burst of aerobic exercise between sets. This strategy will not only let you fit in more exercise into a shorter period of time, since you are resting less, it might also add a little cardiovascular exercise to your strength training regimen.

3. Just as you can make stretching a mindfulness exercise, the same can be done with strength training – feeling your muscles slowly tighten and relax with each repetition.

# 16
# Communication

*"Words are singularly the most powerful force available to humanity. We can choose to use this force constructively with words of encouragement, or destructively using words of despair."*
Yehuda Berg, rabbi

What does communication have to do with relaxation? Whether the setting is home or work, much of our stress centers on dealing with other people. In turn, applying a few simple communication skills will reduce your stress. Not only that, but if your communication skills are sub-par, your co-workers, family, and friends will most likely suffer.

In summary, poor communications skills can lead to a vicious cycle of increasing stress in which people just get angrier and angrier at each other. And then the circle widens – Bob gets in an argument with Sarah and Sarah is upset. Sarah then takes it out on Robin ... and on and on, until your initial, snarky remark ultimately causes World War III.

At its worst, communication can cause hostile stress-inducing environments at home and work. Conversely, at its best, communication causes connection, warmth, and love. When people on their death beds look back on their lives, this type of connection is what they treasure the most. It is arguably what life is about.

*As many people know, training to become a physician is not finished with medical school graduation. Typically, during the last year of medical school, students apply for a residency – further on-the-job training. I concluded my visit to a prestigious family medicine residency with an interview with the program director – a distinguished professor, responsible for not only running this program, but also for creating the preeminent continuing family medicine education course in the United States. Toward the end of the interview, the program director asked me, "How do you think you did in the interview?" I answered, "I think I did well." Therefore, when he asked if I had further questions, it seemed appropriate for me to ask, "How do you think I did in the interview?" The acclaimed senior physician paused briefly and then said, "You seemed very comfortable with yourself."*

*I walked outside of his office, confidant in my superior communication and interview skills. That is, until I looked down and saw that my fly had been wide open during the entire interview. So that is what he meant by my "being comfortable" with myself – having my zipper down during an important job interview.*

## The Basics

**"Communication is a skill that you can learn. It's like riding a bicycle or typing. If you're willing to work at it, you can rapidly improve the quality of every part of your life."**
Brian Tracy, speaker

Prior to recommending specific communications skills, let's start with the basic principles. Of course, zipping up your fly before an important interview may be the first to consider. But there are other basics and that leads us to a psychologist named Carl Rogers, widely regarded as the father of "humanistic" or "client-centered" psychology. Unlike earlier psychologists who emphasized a variety of theories on how the mind worked, Dr. Rogers stressed the importance of human connection. He emphasized three basic principles: Unconditional positive regard or acceptance, empathy, and genuineness. Unconditional positive regard, or acceptance, is illustrated by the following Carl Rogers quote:

*"One of the most satisfying feelings I know —*
*and also one of the most growth – promoting*
*experiences for the other person — comes from my*
*appreciating this individual in the same way that*
*I appreciate a sunset. People are just as wonderful*
*as sunsets, if I can let them be. In fact, perhaps*
*the reason we can truly appreciate a sunset is that*
*we cannot control it. When I look at a sunset, as I*
*did the other evening, I don't find myself saying,*
*'Soften the orange a little on the right-hand corner,*
*and put a little purple along the base, and use a*
*little more pink in the cloud color.'*
*I don't do that. I don't try to control a sunset.*
*I watch it with awe as it unfolds. I like myself best*
*when I can appreciate my staff member, my son,*
*my daughter, my grandchildren,*
*in this same way."*

Unconditional positive regard has two elements:

1. Be mindful as you listen to someone; that is, be present and pay close attention to the other person during the conversation. Author Marge Piercy pointed out, "If you want to be listened to, you should put in time listening." The conversation will be more productive if your partner feels fully heard.

2. Acceptance of a person as he or she is. People have different styles. Some are like a sunset: mellow and easy to be with. Others are like the Rocky Mountains: rough and gruff. The Rocky Mountains can be a beautiful and awe-inspiring place to visit. However, if you are in the mountains and spend all of your time wishing that you were watching a sunset at the beach, you will not be happy. To connect with someone, it helps to let go of your judgments (and thoughts) of how they should be and listen to them as they truly are.

Accepting people as they are and learning to enjoy their individuality does not mean you accept everything they do. As a saying goes, you can "love the sinner without loving the sin." We might wish someone changes in the future and we may even offer feedback to change future behavior. However, in the present, people can only be as they are.

Acceptance also does not require you to spend time with that person. If you are at a zoo, you may see a lion and really admire it but don't jump into its cage. On occasion, one might hear of a woman whose husband repeatedly beats her, but she continues to stay with him because she says she loves him. In this case, it would be better to love from afar.*

The next key component of good communication is empathy.

> **"If there is any great success in life, it lies in the ability to put yourself in the other person's place and to see things from his point of view – as well as your own."**
>
> Henry Ford

Empathy sometimes gets confused with pity, which is very different. With pity, you may look down on another person. With empathy, you put yourself in the other person's shoes. Empathy underlines our commonality. Even if we have not gone through a death in the family, we have all had losses and know what loss feels like. We may never know exactly what another goes through, but we can try to get close. In fact, one of the few good things about our painful times is that they allow us to identify more closely with another's pain. Sometimes, the best training a doctor receives is when he or she, or his or her family member, is a patient.

Where there is an empathetic listener, both people in a conversation benefit. Empathy is not only an effective communication tool but also an effective stress management tool in its own right. When we can try to see life from another's point of view we may notice our own anger, hostility, and stress fading. Empathy allows us to be more patient with friends, family members, and strangers

---

*For brevity, I have oversimplified the predicament that certain abused spouses find themselves in. For further support, contact the National Domestic Violence Hot Line at 1-800-799-SAFE; for hearing-impaired TDD at 1-800-787-3224. For emergencies, dial 911.

we interact with throughout the day, as well as with people whom we've never talked to.

I once had a discussion with a patient with severe emphysema who claimed he was so upset by slow drivers that he'd gone back to smoking. If this same patient had been able to empathize with the predicament of the other drivers, he might not have felt as compelled to jeopardize his health.

In 1995, a man sped through an intersection in Baltimore after the light had turned red. He hit the driver's side of my mother's car and almost killed her. She fractured three ribs on each side, fractured her pelvis, and punctured both lungs. The injured lungs could not function correctly and predisposed her to subsequent life-threatening pneumonia. She spent two months in an intensive-care unit on a breathing machine – unable to talk – and an additional several months recovering. Miraculously, with the help of a dedicated medical team and a lot of prayer, she recovered. But as you might suspect, when she first resumed driving, she was nervous and sometimes drove a little slowly.*

The next time you get annoyed at the driver in front of you, realize that he may have a good reason for his behavior. Perhaps he is lost. Perhaps it is an even more dramatic situation as described above. Empathy allows us to recognize that there are many other stories besides our own.

---

*There is a very legitimate worry about drunk drivers and the high percentage of deadly accidents they cause. I have wondered if a lot of accidents and deaths are also caused by drivers trying to make it through the yellow light. Certainly, many accidents are caused by sleep-deprived drivers.

In addition to its healing potential, there are other practical benefits of empathy. Let's pretend that it's your job to make the schedules for two bosses: Boss A and Boss B. One day, Boss A tells you that you should schedule her appointments every 30 minutes. The next day, Boss B tells you that appointments should be scheduled every hour; therefore, you schedule people every hour. Four days later, Boss A storms into your office and yells, "What an idiot! Can't you do anything right? I gave simple instructions to schedule people every 30 minutes and you couldn't even follow them." There are several ways to respond to this situation:

1. You say to yourself, "Poor me. I always get these unreasonable, awful bosses. I'll probably lose the job." (Let's call this the victim response – not very productive.)

2. You say to your boss, "You think I'm the idiot? You are the stupidest person I've ever met!" (The aggressive response – don't be surprised if you get fired and have trouble getting a good reference letter.)

3. You say to your boss, "Yes, Boss. No problem. I'll do it however you want me to. Sorry to inconvenience you." At the same time you think to yourself, "Well, she wants people scheduled more frequently. Let's see how she likes having them scheduled every 10 minutes." (The passive-aggressive response – may be fun in the short term, but unproductive in the long term.)

---

So, if you have been drinking, don't drive; if you are tired, pull over and rest; and if you see a yellow light, stop if possible. And certainly, do not text while driving. It's too easy to temporarily lose respect for the amount of damage, loss of life, and family pain that can be caused by drivers that are rushed, careless, distracted or drunk.

4. You say to your boss, "I understand why you are upset. If I asked an employee to do something and it looked as if he disregarded my request for no reason, I would be angry as well. However, shortly after you gave your instructions, Boss B told me to schedule people every hour. I assumed you were aware of this. If you and Boss B can decide together on my instructions, I'll be happy to comply." (The empathetic response. Notice how you first empathize with your boss, so she feels acknowledged, and then ask her to empathize with you.)

Genuineness, the third essential component of good communication, follows naturally when unconditional positive regard and empathy are present. It is not genuine to tell someone how wonderful he is while thinking that he is a jerk. However, it is genuine to have a thought that someone is a jerk, let that thought go, and then relate to that person in an empathetic and accepting manner.

With empathy, acceptance, attentiveness, and genuineness, our ordinary conversations can be transformed into something warm, intimate, and beneficial to both parties. Even when the situation is sad, we can have healing conversations that bring us closer.

*Barbara was having a lot of trouble communicating with her 9-year-old daughter Robin. Barbara felt the trouble was that they both had short tempers and would yell at each other. When I asked for more information, I found that Barbara complained that Robin would say things like "All the other mothers spend more time with their daughters."*

*Barbara would argue that it was not true, since she knew that most of the mothers of Robin's friends had full-time jobs. Barbara needed to work full time to make ends meet. I suggested that the next time Robin said, "All the other mothers spend more time with their daughters," Barbara start her response by expressing empathy: "Robin, it sounds as if you are really frustrated that we don't spend more time together." And only after Robin felt understood, then she might go on to say, "I really would like it if we could spend more time together as well. However, I need to work to pay the bills. If you get most of your homework done at your after-school program, when I pick you up we could spend extra time together at the park."*

Can empathy help with the stress of caring for infants and raising young children?

*When our twins were born, we tried to empathize with the newest members of our family. They did not cry to annoy us. If their crying was hard to deal with at 3 a.m., it was important to reframe the situation and to realize that the crying was our children's only way of communicating their needs. We learned to try one strategy after another – feeding? diaper change? sucking? burping? being held? Being put down? – until we satisfied their need.*

Toddlers are in the process of learning to deal with feelings of anger and frustration. One mother, Elizabeth, made the analogy of a toddler's feelings during a tantrum as being similar to the worst case of PMS that could be imagined. Additionally, a toddler has limited language skills to express his desires and frustrations. In essence, it is like having PMS feelings, while most of your words come out garbled and incomprehensible. During tantrums, Elizabeth tries to keep that analogy in mind to help her empathize with her toddler. She then can better understand that her child needs help learning to deal with his intense feelings.

## The Specifics

Now that we've discussed the basic principles, let's explore some more specific communication hints:

1. **Actively listen**. Have you ever spoken to a person who looks past you as you speak and never really hears what you are saying? Bet that made you feel special. Unless you're a ruthless dictator, you really can't force people to attentively listen to you. However, you can control how well you listen to others. And, in turn, if people feel that they are fully heard, they are more likely to hear what you are saying. Former U.S. Secretary of State Dean Rusk said, "One of the best ways to persuade others is with your ears – by listening to them." Even if your goal of the conversation is to persuade another, you'll have little success unless the other person feels understood. Often people will be open to hear your point, only after they are convinced you've fully appreciated theirs. And this whole persuasion thing aside, you'll learn more when you don't act like you already know everything. When a learned rabbi was asked his definition of wisdom, he replied that a wise man knows how to learn from each person he meets. Be mindful when you listen,

and let go of distracting thoughts. When you converse with someone, do your best to learn what that person feels and thinks.

2. **When your goal in a conversation is to win ... you lose.** Think about communication at its best. Do you remember a time when you and another both felt fully understood, when you truly connected? There was no sense that one of you won and the other lost. In a real sense, you both won. When you enter a conversation with the prime goal of being right, much is lost. On the other hand, if your prime goal is to connect and understand, now you're talkin'! And others are listening. Take pride in your ability to communicate, not in your ability to insist on being right.

> *"We must love them both – those whose opinions we share and those whose opinions we reject. For both have labored in the search for truth, and both have helped us in the finding of it."*
>
> Saint Thomas Aquinas

And to make the point a little differently:

> *"To keep your marriage brimming*
> *With love in the marriage cup,*
> *Whenever you're wrong, admit it*
> *Whenever you're right, shut up."*
>
> Ogden Nash, poet

**3. I-statements.** Imagine you're talking with your friend or spouse and they say, "You are inconsiderate!" How do you feel? Perhaps a little defensive? A little annoyed? Now imagine that instead he or she says, "I felt hurt when you insulted me in front of the whole group." Now you might be a little more understanding and a little less defensive. This brings us to the concept of "you-statements" and "I-statements."

When you say, "I feel ..." and go on to describe your feelings, people listen and are less likely to get defensive. Also, people can't effectively argue against a statement about how you feel. On the other hand, statements like, "You should not have acted that way" and "You were an idiot" are likely to elicit arguments and defensiveness.

Below are some more examples. Think of how you'd feel after hearing the I-statement versus the you-statement:

*"You were inconsiderate* by being so late!"
**vs.**
"When I didn't hear from you, *I was afraid* that you might have gotten into an accident. I care a lot about you, so please call the next time you are running late."

"I can't believe *you are eating ice cream again.* You know it's not on your diet!"
**vs.**
*"I really care about you. I'm afraid* that one day you'll have another heart attack and I might lose you. It really worries me when you eat a lot of high-fat foods."

Next is a tricky one. How would you feel if someone said, "I feel that you are domineering." That statement might sound like a feeling, but it is really an opinion. Compare that with "I felt hurt when you did not give me time to express my opinion. I need a moment to let you know what I think about the issue."

In general, if you follow "I feel" with either the word "you" or "that," you're not making the type of I-statement I am recommending. You're not going to make any friends by saying "I feel that you are an idiot!"

*Denise had a difficult time getting along with her sister Alice. I asked for a specific example of one of their conversations:*

*Denise: I was really hurt when you called me fat in front of others.*

*Alice: You always say things like that to me.*

*Denise: I would never do that. You are so inconsiderate.*

*And then an argument and hard feelings ensued.*

*Suggestion of an alternative response for Denise: "I didn't realize that I've said things that have hurt you. If you see that I am doing something like that, let me know right away. I really will try my best not to offend you. I care about you, and hurting you is the last thing that I would want."*

With this alternative response, Denise does not use "you" terms, and she does not insist on winning an argument.

**4. Expressing empathy.** We already covered the importance of empathy. However, even in a fantasy world in which you could completely and totally understand another person, if that dude thinks you don't understand him, there's still a problem. The challenge is not only to understand someone, but to communicate that understanding.

Imagine that you have been struggling with a complex problem. If a friend just quickly volunteers a solution, you might think that he or he has not taken the time to fully understand the problem and is trivializing your struggle. On the other hand, once you knew that your friend understood the problem and its difficulty, you would be more open to his input. Even if he didn't offer any solutions, just knowing you are understood brings its own comfort.

How can you communicate your empathy? Say, "I know how you feel," and you may hear back: "How can you know how I feel?" There may be times when you have undergone a very similar problem. For instance, both you and a friend may have had a parent with Alzheimer's disease. If you are sensitive, discussing your similar struggles may communicate your understanding. Support groups rely on this type of shared understanding.

Whether you share a common situation or not, one of the most effective ways to communicate empathy is to paraphrase. Paraphrasing involves restating what someone says in another form. Paraphrasing does not mean parroting back exactly what someone said. For our purposes, effective paraphrasing is done by condensing or summarizing both the content of what someone said and also their emotional state. After a friend tells you a dozen things that went wrong that day, you might express empathy by saying, "It sounds like a really frustrating day with one problem after another."

In many cases, it is more effective to begin with "That is a stressful situation" before saying, "Just do _____ to fix the problem."

This strategy is important in talking with adults and children. One might say to a young child, "That's silly to be upset about losing that stuffed animal; you have several others." The child is likely to become even more upset because you did not appreciate his or her feelings. Something might not seem important from an adult perspective but it may seem extremely important from the child's perspective. You might do better if you said, "I know you really liked your giraffe. That was upsetting to you to lose it."

Once in a while, people reach an impasse; neither person understands the other's point of view. Instead of fully listening while the other person is talking, each person spends that time planning how to "win" the conversation. Requiring paraphrasing in this type of conversation forces both parties to listen to each other and attempt to empathize.

## Practice

### "TALKING-CUP" EXERCISE

The following exercise can be used to help two people move beyond an impasse in a conversation:

Only one person is allowed to speak at a time. While this person is making a point, he holds an object such as an empty paper cup. Or use an something that can't inflict injury should the disagreement get too heated. After the first person makes his point (hopefully using "I-statements"), the second person must accurately paraphrase the first person's point before she obtains possession of the object and has a turn to make her point. It may take a few attempts to accurately paraphrase a point. When the first person feels it was accurately paraphrased, the object changes hand and it is the second person's chance to make a point and the first person's job to listen and paraphrase it.

5. **It's not always about you.** If you find yourself saying, "I don't deserve to be treated this way," you may indeed be correct. However, how you are treated is often not a consequence of what you do or do not deserve. Rather, it may largely be the consequence of what is going on with the other person. Instead of immediately becoming defensive, try being empathetic to the other's situation and challenges. Be open to learning what may be intentionally or unintentionally contributing to the other's frustration or anger. What is he or she feeling? What does he or she need?

*Peter got home from work one Friday afternoon, after his wife, Lisa, had had a particularly difficult week. It is hard enough to take care of a sick child, but she had been taking care of two sick children that week, when she herself had also been very sick. Understandably, she was in a bad mood when Peter got home. A thoughtful friend of theirs called, and Peter described described how his wife had "ripped his head off" as soon as he got home. Their friend said, "Go put your head back on and help out."*

It is important not to take things too personally. It's better to be less defensive and more empathetic. Give people some slack and "go put your head back on."

6. **Reframing** allows you to listen to comments constructively instead of defensively. It also helps you to find a positive meaning in what others say. One woman recounted an interaction with her loving, but sometimes critical, mother. The woman's fiancé had been a successful businessman, but his luck had changed. His business was bankrupt, and he had also declared personal bankruptcy. When the woman reluctantly revealed the news to her mother, her mother reacted by saying, "You have a knack for finding losers." This statement was very painful to the woman until she reframed it in a positive light. She reasoned that her mother had meant to convey her disappointment since she wanted her daughter to find someone successful and to be happy. Once the woman was able to reframe her mother's initial comment and understand its motivation, she felt better. It is not uncommon for apparently negative comments to be

motivated by caring and concern. Therefore, it often pays to look for the motivation behind a comment.

7. **Clarify.** If you are not sure what the other person's point is, ask for clarification. Communication can be improved by asking for clarification not only of a specific statement, but also about the associated thoughts and feelings.

8. **Listen to both the emotion and the words.** When someone expresses his or her viewpoint in an emotional or loud manner, the tendency is to react by becoming argumentative. Instead of immediately getting argumentative or defensive, take a moment not only to listen to the words but also to consider the emotions implied and expressed. Remember that the intensity of the emotion is a loud signal that the issue is very important to the person with whom you are speaking. Therefore, take some extra time and patience to listen to what he or she is saying.

9. **Nonthreatening:** If at all possible, avoid saying something that could be interpreted as a threat. Most people (probably including yourself) tend to respond negatively to this form of communication. Just imagine your response if someone said, "Do this, or else."

10. **Keep to the Topic.** Do not throw in the kitchen sink. That is, keep to the topic of the current disagreement.

11. **Keep an internal locus of control.** Do not blame others for your emotions. Your conversation will be more productive if you avoid blame in general. Using "I" statements can help you do this.

12. **Sometimes writing issues down can help.** Usually, it is best to address a concern as soon as you can. However, there are times when someone is not available to communicate or you need time to compile your thoughts. When you find yourself reviewing a conversation again and again in your head, list the main points of the conversation on paper. With your concerns on paper, you might no longer feel the need to rehearse the conversation continually in your mind. Instead of writing the concerns on paper, you could also type them on your computer. However, don't send any emails without adequate forethought. Those points you wrote down when you were angry at 2 a.m. may no longer seem as valid in the light of day. Sending a poorly thought-out email may really add to your stress.

# 17
# Communication Part 2

## Feedback

*One of my English teachers, Ms. Backfeed, told a story of her college days. Some guy sent her a love note. Ms. Backfeed, gave him back the note ... after correcting the grammar and spelling with her red marker.*

In general, there are better ways to give feedback than using a red marker on a love note. Hopefully, Ms. Backfeed's unfortunate would-be amore had a good sense of humor. My experience with college grammar correction was not quite as painful. When I was a freshman, an upperclassman would frequently correct my grammar. Eventually, I said in frustration, "What are you, a grammatician?" He answered, "No, I'm a grammarian."

Often, it's best to just accept another's behavior. After all, in this moment people can only be as they are. Yet there are times when it would be great to change another's future behavior. If you don't happen to have a magic wand, how might you accomplish this?

Perhaps insulting someone? Would that change someone's behavior? I would argue that it may indeed change a person's behavior ... in exactly the wrong direction. Call someone a rude jackass and you expect them to be less rude? That's like dropping a barbell on your toe and expecting it to feel good.

As covered in an earlier chapter, when Dr. Sidney Farber found that folate caused leukemia patients to die, his solution was to use an anti-folate drug. So let's look at what makes a good insult and do the opposite. Remember the goal of an insult is to make someone feel bad. The goal of feedback is to influence behavior and the goal of negative feedback is to make it less likely someone repeats an undesired behavior.

An insult such as "You are a complete idiot!" is a demeaning comment about a general trait. Therefore, good feedback:

- Should not be insulting or demeaning.

- Should refer to a person's behavior rather than a trait. For instance, instead of "You are clumsy," effective feedback might be "When you use your large drill, be sure to use both hands and use your left hand for the lever." Similarly, calling someone rude is usually less effective than asking him or her to let you finish a story before interrupting.

- Feedback should be as specific as possible. Instead of saying "You do careless work," you could explain which specific project needed improvement and what specific improvements were needed. This precise information will be much more useful in preventing a similar mistake in the future.

Additional hints on giving effective feedback:

- Feedback needs to be understandable. Unless both parties are very familiar with jargon and technical terms, it's best avoided. Even when you don't use jargon, make sure to make your message clear.

- Feedback should be well-timed. If you're being criticized, do you want a large audience? I'm guessing your answer is "not so much." In general, negative feedback should be given individually. (Whereas sometimes it may appropriate to give positive feedback in front of a group.) Feedback should usually be given as soon after the event as possible. It's far from ideal to think you're performing just fine and then receive negative comments when it's too late to change – too late to change, but not too late to be annoyed. Therefore, give feedback as soon after an event as possible.

- Pick your battles. Giving feedback soon after an event will and should increase the frequency of feedback. However, let's not go nuts with this – too frequent negative feedback can be interpreted as nitpicking. If you give continuous negative feedback, morale will likely drop and all your comments may be ignored. This is where the art comes in: Giving feedback frequently enough so that it is well-timed, but avoiding non-stop feedback on relatively unimportant matters.

- Prior to giving feedback, it is often helpful to express your empathy. As mentioned earlier, once people feel understood, they will be more open to feedback.

- No one likes to hear feedback only when things go wrong. Does someone need to win the Nobel Prize before you say "Good job"? Positive feedback is given to make it more likely someone repeats a desired behavior. A good hint for giving positive feedback, whether it be in raising children or talking to co-workers, is to catch someone doing something right. Don't wait for a heroic act. With young children, you might really need to be creative with that positive feedback: "You've been playing so well with your brother for the last 30 seconds." (For those of you who plan to have children but don't yet, and think I'm joking about the 30 seconds – hee hee hee.) Positive feedback can be as effective as, or even more effective than, negative feedback. Positive feedback has an added bonus: The next time negative feedback is given, it is likely to be received more willingly and less defensively. No one who is working hard likes to hear only negative comments. All of the preceding points about negative feedback are applicable to positive feedback as well – make feedback specific and about a behavior, not a trait. "You are conscientious" is a nice compliment, and compliments definitely have their place. However, telling someone the specific behavior you liked is more likely to increase the continuation of that behavior.

> **"Everyone wants to be appreciated,**
> **so if you appreciate someone,**
> **don't keep it a secret."**
>
> Mary Kay Ash
> Founder, Mary Kay Cosmetics

- Feedback is more effective when someone feels fully understood before the feedback is delivered. Therefore, prior to giving feedback, it is often important to empathize and communicate that empathy.

• If you want to make sure the feedback was understood, you might want to ask the other person to summarize what you said. Take ownership of the communication. Obviously, don't say, "Since you're such a bonehead, you better repeat what I just told you." Instead, say something like: "I'm not sure I did a good job giving you feedback. Let me double check that you understood it. What's your understanding of what to do with the project?" If the person heard the feedback in terms of a trait, you can restate it in terms of the specific behavior.

*Wendy was very frustrated about the performance of her employees. She complained that when she would ask them to do a task, it would often be done incorrectly. I asked if she had checked with her employees to see why they were not getting the job done. She said that she had asked. However, what she had asked was, "Did you not listen to me, or are you just not able to do the job?" I asked Wendy to consider checking into the problem in a way that would be less demeaning to her employees. I emphasized that it was more important to communicate effectively than to try to "be right." She had more success when she took care not to be patronizing or insulting. She sincerely said, "It seems I am not effectively communicating what needs to be done. Is there a different or new way that I could discuss the assignment so you understand it better?" Once she did give the instructions, she could check on whether her employees understood them. For instance, she*

*could say, "I'm still not sure I am doing a good*
*job getting my message across. This information*
*might be confusing. To make sure I did get*
*the message across, could you please tell*
*me your understanding of what we discussed*
*before you get started on the project?"*

## Receiving Feedback

An old story tells of an arrogant student asking to be a
disciple of a wise Zen master. The master asks the student if he would like some tea. When the student says,
"Yes, please," his cup is filled and then overfilled. The tea
flows from the rim of the cup to the table and then to the
floor. When the student protests, the master explains that
he cannot teach someone whose cup is already full. Sometimes we are so eager to prove that we know the truth, we
can't really hear (or benefit from) feedback. There is most
always room for improvement, but if we are not open to
feedback, our performance will likely stagnate.

There is skill in receiving feedback as well as in giving
it. The problem is not all seven billion people on Earth
have read this book, so there is a lot of poorly delivered
feedback out there. Even poorly delivered feedback may
contain a useful message. If someone offers feedback to
you that is not specific or is about a trait rather than a
behavior, you may be tempted to get defensive and
perhaps even angry. Before reacting with anger,
consider asking for clarification. Is there a specific behavior that should be improved? Also, do not listen only
to the person's words. What is the feeling behind the
communication? What is the need that the person may

be expressing? By asking these questions and by asking for clarification when needed, you can avoid feeling insulted. You can also ascertain if the feedback contains useful advice.

We've all been subject to nasty criticism. At times, I have been able to let go of my initial defensiveness and pain and then distill some useful feedback out of a rude comment. Sometimes finding the kernel of useful information takes a bit of imagination and usually a double dose of humility. There are other instances when the comment is pure insult and no useful information can be found even with a microscope. Whenever you receive a less-than-polite remark, remember what Theodore Roosevelt said:

> *"It is not the critic who counts; not the man who points out how the strong man stumbles, or where the doer of deeds could have done them better. The credit belongs to the man who is actually in the arena, whose face is marred by dust and sweat and blood; who strives valiantly; who errs .... [And] if he fails, at least fails while daring greatly."*

*Ann was getting frustrated with a co-worker, Robin. At most of their group meetings, Robin would seem to nitpick Ann's performance. This was incredibly stressful for Ann. On my suggestion, Ann reframed the situation and realized that Robin, at times, actually had given some useful feedback. When Ann thought about it, she realized that what she really resented was that the feedback was given in a group setting. Instead of being angry at Robin, she thanked Robin for the feedback that was useful. She then requested that Robin give her feedback privately. Thereafter, Ann and Robin got along better, and Ann could actually use some of Robin's feedback instead of just growing annoyed at her nitpicking.*

And here is one of the most important questions: "How skillfully have you delivered feedback to yourself?" Let's say something goes wrong and you tell yourself, "I'm so stupid!" What kind of grade would you give that piece of self-feedback? It's demeaning, about a trait (not a behavior), and is not specific. A bit better would be, "Next time I'm in the wilderness, I won't use that three-leafed plant for toilet paper." Whether you talk to yourself or others, effective feedback will make your day go better.

---

### Relax on the Run

### SKILLFUL FEEDBACK

Whether talking to others or thinking to yourself, remember to make your feedback about a specific behavior. (It should not be about a trait and should not be demeaning.)

---

## Take Some Time

*Author and communication expert Marshall Rosenberg tells the story of taking a long pause before responding to one of his sons. He was struggling to find the words to communicate in a thoughtful, nonaggressive manner. His son, becoming impatient with the pause, said, "Daddy, it's taking you so long to talk." Rosenberg*

*responded, "Let me tell you what I can say quickly:*
*'Do it my way or I'll kick your butt.'" His son said,*
*"Take your time, Dad. Take your time."*

Instead of reflexively acting, sometimes we need to take a second or two (or much longer) to come up with an effective way of communicating. It can be a struggle as we think about one insult or one "you" statement after another. Then, finally, we find the right words. Especially as we are first learning a new way to communicate, we may really need to pause to think about how we would like to respond. Old habits take some effort to break. However, if you want to improve your relationships at home and work, it is well worth it.

---

**Practice**

## THE SLOW RESPONSE

The next time you are about to respond during a stressful conversation, take the time to think about your answer. Try to follow the communication guidelines expressed in this chapter when you do respond.

---

## Listen With Another Set of Ears

In his workshops, Marshall Rosenberg has a unique way of illustrating two different styles of communication. He uses the jackal as a symbol of aggressive communication and the giraffe as a symbol of what he calls non-violent communication (NVC). Then he can visually illustrate different ways of hearing by putting on different sets of fake ears. Putting on his jackal ears, he can show how a comment may cause an angry or sad reaction.

## PUTTING ON NEW EARS

When someone else makes a statement and you are just starting to get annoyed, can you (figuratively of course) put on a new set of ears? Can you listen not just to the words but to what feelings and needs are behind the words?

When he puts on the giraffe ears, he not only listens to the words but also tries to find the feelings and the needs that the other person is expressing. The image of actually putting on another set of ears drives home the point that there are different ways of hearing.

I used to have puppet giraffe ears that I could put on my head to illustrate the concept of non-violent communication. When one of my sons was around 9 years old, he tore one of the ears off. The irony, of course, was that I couldn't really yell at him about destroying my non-violent communication toy. If he was going to break something, he chose well.

When the Buddha was about to obtain enlightenment, Mara shot 1,000 arrows at him. The arrows fell to his feet as flowers. Keep this image in mind the next time you think that someone is shooting verbal arrows at you.

## The Art of Apology

Have you ever gone to apologize to someone and epically failed? You were trying to smooth things out, but before you knew it, an intense argument resulted – your attempt worked as well as putting out a fire with gasoline. What is the explanation?

Let's review a scenario: You realize that you've acted inappropriately and go to apologize. Perhaps you feel bad. It is understandable and very natural to want to be understood and to want to describe why you acted the way you did. Here is the problem: Your attempt to be understood could easily be misunderstood as an attempt to justify your actions. "I'm sorry. I shouldn't have done ABC, but I did it because you did XYZ." And then the argument proceeds: "I did XYZ, because you did ..."

How might you increase your chance of successfully apologizing? First off, do you need to say anything to explain your motivations, or is it better to just apologize? Often, a simple apology without explanation works best. For instance, you might say, "I'm sorry. I won't do it again." Of course, if you promise not to repeat a behavior, you need to keep your promise.

In certain circumstances, you may feel it important to explain your actions.

Maybe you feel being better understood will help resolve the problem. Perhaps it will prevent future problems. If you feel the explanation is important, be mindful of the tendency for people to misinterpret your intention. Clearly state how you were wrong and apologize. Then you can clarify that you want to explain why you acted inappropriately. Remember to explain yourself with "I" statements. For instance, you might say, "I'm sorry. I really acted inappropriately. I am not justifying my actions, but I want to explain why I acted that way. It was a very long day at work. I was already frustrated and became more frustrated being reminded of the tasks I'd forgotten. I was way off base and apologize." Your apology does not need to be lengthy; just be aware of the pitfall of the "justifying apology."

If the matter for which you are apologizing for is more significant, the process of apology may need to be more involved. The Jewish tradition includes several steps of an apology. These include, after apologizing for the action (or inaction), asking how the offense affected the other person. I recommend that if the aggrieved party is willing to share this information, you should do your best to empathize with the harmed party and should try to express that empathy (keeping in mind the ideas discussed earlier in the chapter such as mindful listening and paraphrasing). The next step is asking the injured party if there is anything that you can do to help, and if possible and reasonable, do that action. Once that injured party is understood and action is done to remedy the problem, the chance of healing may increase.

## Assertiveness

> **"You can't have everything.**
> **Where would you put it?"**
> Steven Wright, comedian

And it follows that you can't do it all. Where would you find the time? We are often asked to do a variety of tasks, and for some of us, a "yes" comes out of our mouths as reflexively as swatting a mosquito. Never mind the thousand other things on your plate; you just agreed to a whole smorgasbord of extra obligations. It is important to be productive and get things done. It is important to do your share of the work. Sometimes it's more than your share, but everything? Really?

At one time or another, most of us have trouble saying "No." What motivates this tendency to be a yes-aholic? Often, it is an overdeveloped need to be liked. Yet, if we speak with honesty, kindness, wisdom, and tact, that compulsion to be liked can take a back seat. As Mahatma Gandhi said, "A 'no' uttered from the deepest conviction is better and greater than a 'yes' merely uttered to please, or what is worse, to avoid trouble."

Being able to honestly express your desires, that is being assertive, is an essential communication skill. Assertiveness should, in no way, imply being aggressive, obnoxious, or rude. Being assertive starts by being true to yourself – following your own sense of integrity and morality instead of blindly trying to win others' approval.

*Henry was performing well at work, but he found himself increasingly busy and stressed. As soon as he finished one project, he was assigned two more. Before he knew it, he was working 70 to 80 hours a week, and other areas of his life were suffering. He came to me complaining of palpitations and anxiety. Henry finally realized that it was rare to find a boss who would start a conversation by saying, "Take it easy; you've worked too hard already." When Henry voiced his desires in a polite, yet assertive, way, his boss was more than willing to accommodate Henry's request for a decreased workload. The palpitations decreased, and Henry had the chance to develop other parts of his life – including a new relationship.*

Let's look at the above example more closely. Henry had several options:

1. Give in and accept any added work his boss would give him (passive response).

2. Angrily call his boss inconsiderate (aggressive response).

3. Politely, yet firmly, advise his boss that his plate was already full with other tasks (assertive response).

Notice how each of the following assertive responses might be appropriate, so Henry could have some time off work:

- "I'm already busy with two other projects, so I don't think that I'll have time for the new project."

- "I'm doing the Smith and Jones project now, and I need to be home by 6 p.m. If you would like me to work on the new project, I'll have to postpone the others. Which project would you prefer that I complete today?" We cannot count on a boss, co-worker, or spouse to automatically try to decrease our stress load. It is essential to realize that if we don't speak up for ourselves, often no one will.

## The Clerk Is Not a Jerk

I remember, many years ago, reading a book that espoused the saying "The clerk is a jerk." What the author meant was that if you want to get something of value from a store, such as a refund, you should seek the manager and not just settle for a negative response from a store salesperson or clerk. It may be true that if you do not get satisfaction from a salesperson, talking with the manager might be helpful. However, far too often people do not treat staff members at a place of business with respect. As the saying goes, "You catch a lot more flies with honey than with vinegar."

When you treat people with respect and a caring attitude, you will accomplish much more, and both of the parties involved will be less frustrated. You can always ask to speak to a supervisor later, but you may be surprised by what can be accomplished by being pleasant and nonthreatening to other employees first. Keep this in mind, too, when talking to people on the phone. It is often too easy to forget that there is another real person on the other end of the line.

## Summary

Throughout this chapter, we have discussed a variety of communication skills. By effectively implementing these skills, you will improve your relationships with people in all aspects of your life. If you practice acceptance, empathy, genuineness and assertiveness, your life will become less stressful and more fulfilled.

---

**Practice**

### COMMUNICATION SKILLS:

List ways you can improve your communication at work and home.

1. _____

2. _____

3. _____

# 18

# Anger and Frustration

I have yet to hear: "It's been such a stressful day. I think I need to take a break from that and get frustrated." Or: "What a day. Can't wait to kick back and get really angry!" Frustration and anger are not relaxing in the least – and not very healthy. We all get angry on occasion, but people who are angry much of the time are more likely to get heart attacks. As the Buddha said thousands of years before modern day cardiovascular research: "Holding onto anger is like holding on to a hot coal with the intent of throwing it at someone else; you are the one that gets burned." Anger can also be destructive to our relationships, resulting in damaged friendships, troubled work environments, broken families and, in extreme cases, violence.

There are a variety of methods to reduce anger and frustration, some of which overlap with relaxation techniques we've already discussed. We also have brand-spanking-new material to cover and even the previously mentioned techniques can be further customized and refined to deal with anger and frustration.

For our first hints in dealing with anger, it makes sense to listen to a guy who got the Nobel Peace Prize – the Dalai Lama. The country of Tibet was invaded by China in 1949. By some estimates, 6,000 Tibetan temples were destroyed and a million Tibetans died as a result of the Chinese occupation. The Dalai Lama is the spiritual leader of the Tibetan Buddhists. Yet the Dalai Lama did not seem to harbor anger toward the Chinese. His reasoning: "They have taken everything from us; should I let them take my mind as well?"

The Dalai Lama realized that if he were to harbor anger and resentment against the Chinese, he, not the Chinese, would be giving up peace of mind. The Dalai Lama continues to lobby for the Tibetan people, but without anger dominating his mind.

How do we deal with our anger? One of the most effective methods is mindfulness. Fighting the anger and wishing it away can just make us angry about being angry. As discussed in depth in earlier chapters, when we welcome our present-moment emotions, thoughts, and sensations, the next moment brings a new experience.

## More About Empathy

Especially relevant to reducing anger and frustration is empathy. Henry Wadsworth Longfellow said: "If we could read the secret history of our enemies, we should find in each man's life sorrow and suffering enough to disarm all hostility." Perhaps not always, but most often, if we could really see the world through another's eyes, our anger would disappear.

Movies, plays, and even books provide wonderful entertainment. However, they have another role in our society. A good show can provide insight into another's perspective. As we sit munching chips on our couch, we can see the world through the eyes of someone on the other side of the planet. We might learn the perspective of someone of another gender, race, religion, occupation ,or sexual orientation. In fact, the end of slavery may have been hastened by Harriet Beecher Stowe's book *Uncle Tom's Cabin* which helped to change the cultural attitude regarding slavery. Movies such as *Remember the Titans* and *42* showed people the effects of racism. Television shows such as *Glee* may have been partially responsible for society's evolving acceptance of gay relationships. In all of these cases and many others, people were able see life through others' eyes and thereby increase their empathy.

Imagine if, when annoyed with a friend, we could hire Steven Spielberg with a $100 dollar budget to instantly make a film showing our friend's perspective. He could include all the relevant background – from childhood relationships to what happened ten minutes prior to the interaction. We could watch how we came across, not from our perspective, but how it looked to another.

Not only would you see the background material that helped shape your friend's viewpoint, you might see that how you think you came across was off base. That time when you knew that you were just speaking a tad loudly – you might be surprised to hear your scream topping the 100 decibels. What you had thought was a polite request may end up sounding more like an abusive barrage of epithets.

The bottom line is our interpretation of an interaction is colored by our preconceived notions, and the other person's viewpoint is colored by their preconceived notions. The ability to view the world through another's eyes is arguably the most important tool for dealing with anger and frustration.

Unfortunately, we can't instantly produce a movie to help us understand our friends and colleagues. However, we can use our imagination and, thus, strengthen our skills in empathy.

## USE YOUR MEMORY

Sometimes, it doesn't take an elaborate imagination to empathize – it just takes your memory. If you are fuming about someone cutting you off on the freeway, remember when you mistakenly cut someone else off. If I start getting annoyed by someone not letting me into a traffic lane, I can remember a time when I was in dense traffic in Washington, D.C. Although I wouldn't usually let another driver in front, in this case, I wanted to keep on my brother-in-law's tail so I wouldn't get lost. So now if someone won't let me into a lane, I think back to the time when I was scared of getting lost

## USE YOUR IMAGINATION

When you are frustrated or angry with another person, try to imagine a movie that presents that person's viewpoint including all the background information and how he or she interpreted your interaction. Then see what you learn. Keep in mind that you might not act the same way the other did, but perhaps you can now understand the person better, and by doing so, be less angry.

## Humor

*"Laughter is a form of internal jogging.*
*It moves your organs around.*
*It enhances respiration.*
*It is an igniter of great expectations."*

Norman Cousins, author

Another way to mitigate frustration is with a little humor. Our sense of humor can help carry us through those times that might otherwise be much more difficult.

To develop your biceps, you need to work out hard at the gym. To develop your sense of humor, watch funny movies, read funny books or check out some jokes on the Internet, which is just the kind of training I like – fun and easy. ("No, I'm not goofing off. I'm training my sense of humor.") If you're up to it, tell a few jokes.

*Once I was traveling to give a lecture. The plane was late, and everyone else's luggage came off before ours. Somewhere across town, there were several hundred people in a rented hall waiting for me to give a talk – perhaps on the importance of being on time – and it was getting later and later. Finally, our luggage started to arrive ... One suitcase had sprung open, and clothes were spread all over the conveyer belt. Another piece of luggage was obviously damaged. The people traveling with me were more and more upset. Finally I said, "Relax, this is funny. In a few weeks we'll be telling stories about tonight and laughing about it. If it'll be funny then it's funny now." And we started looking at the situation as if it were a Woody Allen movie. When some of the luggage didn't arrive, we smiled. When the car rental company didn't have our reservation (or cars), we laughed. When we heard there was a taxi strike, we howled.*

John-Roger, author

Title that problem in the kitchen "Abbott and Costello Meet the Waffle Maker." Muse about the computer problem as if you were in a Marx Brothers movie. I put a postcard in the mailbox, but forgot it needed a stamp – "Laurel and Hardy and the Mail."

When you make a mistake, see if you can find the humor, then laugh, learn and move on. In one moment, the tears might be flowing or we might be shaking with stress. Then, suddenly, by seeing the humor in the situation, we can laugh. Remember, if it will be funny in 10 years, it's funny now.

*People were very stressed at Sally's workplace. It seemed that much of the staff was on vacation in August. The remaining staff members were therefore getting behind in processing orders. As they got further behind, they had to respond to more and more phone calls about the late orders. These further delayed the process. Several hour-long and seemingly irrelevant work meetings made the situation worse. Sally designed a sign for the bulletin board that said, "Seven-hour meeting today to discuss why the work is backlogged." The humor seemed to draw the staff together and lighten the mood, though Sally is currently unemployed (just joking.)*

## Forgiveness

*"The weak can never forgive.*
*Forgiveness is the*
*attribute of the strong."*

Mahatma Gandhi

Every major religion advocates forgiveness. For those who don't believe in any formal religion, then you certainly believe in the one true source of all knowledge – namely Wikipedia, of course. According to Wikipedia, those "who forgive are happier and healthier than those who hold resentments." Our relationships are too important to let grudges over old problems predominate our mind and twist up our insides.

I remember a time, many years ago, when someone really read me the riot act. And for once, I didn't deserve it. At that time, my wife and I were in the feeding, changing diapers and constant monitoring marathon otherwise known as having twin babies. When I wasn't working at work, I was working at home. My wife and I knew how hard both of us were working. However, when someone else loudly rebuked me for not pulling my weight during a rare vacation, I was sensitive, angry, and felt like holding the grudge of all grudges.

And yet, I remembered another time with another person. I had yelled at that person unfairly. As soon as I did, I realized my error. My apology was not enough to mollify the situation, and it took awhile for me to earn forgiveness. I saw similar situations from both sides. It was clear to me that our emotions are like the weather. At times, anger comes in storms; during these storms people may unleash torrents of unwarranted, unwise and downright rude accusations. People often say things they don't truly mean in the midst of the storm of anger. In such cases, keeping a grudge against someone is like spending a sunny day being upset because yesterday was stormy.

We have all acted inappropriately at one time or another. We also have had people treat us inappropriately. They may have said or done something that was really off base. Being able to forgive is one of the most important qualities we can have in our relationships and for our own health.

---

**Relax on the Run**

### ANGER STORM

Use the analogy that anger is like a storm. Even when people care about each other, once in a while we all lose our temper. The anger can blow into our lives with the ferocity of a hurricane. However, when the storm of anger is over, it is over.

---

When it seems hard to forgive, consider using a meditative approach:

---

**Practice**

## FORGIVENESS MEDITATION

In this meditation, we recognize that all people, knowingly and unknowingly, have at times harmed themselves and others. Get comfortable and close your eyes. Spend a few moments focused on your breath. Then say to yourself, "May I be forgiven for any harm I have caused others either knowingly or unknowingly." Then go on to say to yourself, "May I be forgiven for any harm I have caused myself either knowingly or unknowingly." Finally, say, "I forgive others for any harm they have committed against me, knowingly or unknowingly." When repeating these phrases, you may notice a decrease in your tendency to get stuck in feelings of anger, as well as a corresponding decrease in your stress. This meditation can be done in anywhere from two to 20 minutes.

---

## Don't Ignore the Positive

Ah, the days of a brand-new relationship with unbridled adoration! Any faults with your date are as invisible as a clean glass window pane. There is plenty of time to discover imperfections, but initially the Windex of infatuation cleans them from your sight.

When you are angry, your outlook could not be more different – it is not the faults that are invisible; it is the good qualities that cannot be seen. No positive attribute can be detected through the thunderclouds of anger.

Every time you repeat to yourself or others all the injustices and faults, it further stokes the flames of anger. And the angrier you get, the less likely you see any redeeming feature.

Remembering and listing the virtues of a friend or family member will give you a truer, more accurate picture of that person and thus reduce the anger.

---

**Practice**

## LIST THE POSITIVE

When you are angry with someone, go out of your way to list the person's positive traits. Also list times or circumstances when he or she has been kind, thoughtful, caring, hardworking, attentive, etc.

1. _____
2. _____
3. _____
4. _____
5. _____

---

## Anger as Motivation

Yet another way to deal with anger is to channel your feelings productively. That is, use the feelings to benefit your own, or another's, well-being. If you smoke, for example, you could use your anger over the hold cigarettes have on you to give you the strength to quit smoking.

Few experiences in life are more emotionally difficult than a parent dealing with the death of a child. How can anyone deal with such anger and grief? In several instances, parents have done something productive with that anger. After Candace Lightner's daughter was killed by a drunk driver, Ms. Lightner started the organization Mothers Against Drunk Driving. More recently, two of my friends lost their son to a drunk driver. Of course, they join a chorus of voices against drunk driving, but the major drive of their work has been to keep alive their son's passion and purpose – improving communication toward the goal of a lasting peace between Israel and Palestine (www.avischaeferfund.org/). Whether these and other parents sought to solve the problem that caused their child's death, or worked to keep their child's mission and purpose alive, their brave, non-violent work not only gives them some comfort, it also makes the world better for the rest of us. Even when an event is not as devastating as the loss of a child, using anger (and/or grief) as a motivation may be of benefit.

## Language and Anger

"That which we call a rose, by any other name would smell as sweet," … or so said or so said Juliet Capulet in Shakespeare's "Romeo and Juliet." However, if Romeo had a different last name, the story of Romeo and Juliet might have turned out quite differently. Our words and language are extremely important. Even in our thoughts, the words we chose can make a big difference in how we feel.

In an earlier chapter, we covered the importance of an internal locus of control. I explained that saying "You made me sad" or "I am sad because you are late" implies an external locus of control. That language gives you only one choice on how to feel. If you want to have a more internal locus of control, you might say, "You were late and I was sad."

There is another type of phrase unique to anger. We don't say, "I'm sad at him" or "I'm happy at her." However, we do say, "I'm angry at him." What's the implication of those words – he caused the anger. You were just standing around, minding your own business, and he forced you to be angry. You had no choice in the matter.

How can you deal with your anger if you blame someone else for it? So, instead of saying, "I'm angry at him," it's better to say, "I'm angry." We can even do better than the phrase "I'm angry." By using the common language convention of "I am angry," we imply that the emotion defines us. Instead of "I am Jay Winner, I am angry." Obviously, there is more to us than our current emotion, but you wouldn't surmise that from the phrases "I am angry" or "I am sad." More accurate might be: "I notice anger" or "There is sadness." Then you can mindfully notice the emotion with curiosity and interest. This applies to all emotions, but it is especially important with anger. In day-to-day life, it is impossible to never say or think phrases like "I am angry." However, being aware of what you are saying and thinking may help to rephrase your language.

Relax on the Run

## MODIFY YOUR LANGUAGE

Next time you think either, "I'm angry because the
____" or "He made me angry," or "I'm angry at
him," try restating the phrase to: "He did ___ and
I notice anger." (You can use the same type of
phrasing to describe another emotion such as sadness.) Mindfully notice the anger and any associated physical sensations and thoughts. Then mindfully
pay attention to a few breaths. Do you notice any
difference in how you feel? Is there any change in
the intensity of the anger?

## Conclusion

Anger can rob you of your relaxation and health. By
empathizing, forgiving, recalling people's positive traits,
and being mindful of our language, we can reduce anger
and frustration.

# 19

# Less Stress Decision-Making

Crouching behind the delicate fern, sweat dripping from his forehead, heart pounding in his chest, then charging the large beast, Caveman Zock clutched his heavy spear. He did not weigh the pros and cons of the attack nor did he ponder the ethics of the hunt – he was implored to act by the gnawing hunger in his gut.

Jump ahead a million years to the present day: sweat dripping from his forehead, heart pounding in his chest, hunting for his food, Zach clutched his heavy shopping cart. Unlike Zock, Zach's life is in no immediate danger, but nevertheless, he feels some stress. He looks down at the word "bread" on the grocery list and ponders his 60 different choices; "soup" – 120 choices; "cereal" – 160 choices; and so on. The world of plenty means the world of plenty decisions. Life-threatening danger and few choices have been replaced by rare danger and countless choices. Even if you don't get stressed at the supermarket, certainly some decisions put you on edge. Where will you live? What job will you take? Whom will you marry? From a background of a thousand smaller daily choices, the occasional large decision arises – like a wharf buffeted by innumerable small choppy waves before being slammed by a tsunami.

Currently, it is not essential that most of us bone up on our spear-throwing technique, but we may need some instruction when it comes to making good decisions with minimal stress.

## Depressurizing Decision-Making

There are multiple effective decision-making strategies, but before we get there, it's useful to focus on lowering the general tension surrounding decisions. If you want to play catch with an overinflated water balloon and not get wet, it makes sense to first untie the knot and take a little water out. In the same way, if you want to make a decision and not stress out, it may make sense to first depressurize the choice with some of the following strategies.

Obviously, not all strategies will be appropriate for a particular decision, but each of them will be suited to some of the decisions that will come your way.

1. Keep in mind that most decisions are not permanent. If you try something and don't like it, you can often reconsider. For some decisions, such as your brand of toothpaste, changing your mind only costs a few bucks; for others, such as your choice of job or residence, changing may be a real inconvenience costing significant time and money; and for still other decisions, such as your choice to have a child, there is no turning back. For the decisions that aren't permanent, keeping that fact in mind may be your first pressure-relief valve.

2. Ask yourself, "Will this decision matter in 10 years?" An answer of "no" may decrease your tension. If "yes" – there are other strategies.

3. Are you struggling with a particular decision? Remind yourself: If a decision is hard to make, usually both choices compare closely in their virtues, so you can't go too wrong either way. After all, if one choice

were much better than the other, the decision would be easy.

4. Remember the concept of internal locus of control. Our happiness and peace of mind will be most influenced by internal factors such as our attitudes and our willingness to focus on the present. We probably can be happy or sad whether we live in Kansas or California, or whether we go to one college or another. We can frequently view our decisions as two alternatives that we could be happy with, as opposed to thinking that all of our happiness depends on the right decision.

## Decision-Making Strategies

*"When you come to a fork in the road, take it."*

Yogi Berra

Once you've decreased your anxiety over the decision, you can employ the following decision-making skills to further decrease your stress, and, hopefully, to help you make a better choice.

*"Half the worry in the world is caused by people trying to make decisions before they have sufficient knowledge on which to base a decision."*

Dean Hawkes

1. As the Dean Hawkes quote implies, doing the necessary research is important. For instance, a book or the Internet may have information that could help with your decision. Be creative in where to look for advice. Ultimately, the decision may be yours, but seeking the advice of others or discussing the options with others can be helpful. Seek someone who is an expert in the field or someone who has had to make a similar decision. You can also discuss the decision with other people who will be affected by its outcome. Some of the people to consider consulting include your family, friends, your co-workers, a counselor, a member of the clergy, or a doctor. President Woodrow Wilson said, "I not only use all the brains that I have, but all that I can borrow."

2. Make a list of pros and cons. Sometimes decision-making is easier when the advantages and disadvantages of each course of action are on paper. Writing the issues on paper or computer will also decrease the tendency to argue the points over and over in your head.

3. At times, the best course of action is sitting with or sleeping on a decision, rather than worrying. Have you ever struggled with a decision and then suddenly something happens or an idea occurs to you and the best choice becomes clear? This is a common phenomenon. If a decision needs to be made now, don't procrastinate. However, time is frequently available to consider the options.

Instead of spending this time worrying, acknowledge that certain choices may become clearer on their own with a little time. Give yourself permission to sleep on or sit with a decision. (Of course, in the meantime, you will do the necessary research, make your list of pros and cons, etc.)

4. In times of extreme emotional turmoil, it may be best, if possible, to postpone important decisions. For instance, when faced with the recent loss of a loved one, you may find it difficult to rationally weigh the pros and cons of a complicated decision. Sometimes decisions cannot be postponed, but if it is possible to postpone a difficult choice during a difficult time, it may be wise.

5. Brainstorming on your own or with another person can be helpful. If you have two obvious choices, brainstorming will likely produce additional ideas. The first step is to come up with as many options as you can, no matter how impractical they might seem. You could ask a friend or group of friends, co-workers, family members, experts or support group to help. Sometimes you will try to brainstorm and only get a drizzle; other times, you might get a flood of ideas. Afterward, you can critically analyze each choice to come up with a smaller, more practical list that may include more than your initial two.

6. Focusing on the values involved in the decision and then weighing those values can be helpful. For instance, some decisions may involve the choice between a job with a higher salary and another that pays less but would be more fulfilling in other

ways. Considering the 40 or more hours per week
you may be at your job, a more fulfilling one may
be more important. However, if earning less means
more difficulty actually putting food on the table,
the additional fulfillment might not be as important.

7. The importance of integrity cannot be overem-
phasized. Don't waste your time feeling guilty. To
quote Abraham Lincoln, "When I do good, I feel
good. When I do bad, I feel bad. That's my religion."
Make the decision you can be proud of, and feel
good about it. With certain decisions, you simply
know what is right. Do it. Think about what your
guiding principles are. For example, "Do not do
any harm, and if possible, try to help others." If
you are religious, consider what you think God
would want you to do. Alternatively, you might ask
yourself, "What course of action would I be proud
to discuss with my children?"

8. Pretend you have made one of the choices, and ask
yourself, "How do I feel?" Now pretend you have
made the other choice and ask the same question.
This may be one way to access your "gut feeling" or
intuition.

9. Sometimes a decision is more difficult when there is
a lot of static in our minds. If your mind seems to be
racing, meditate, take a walk, or practice a
walking meditation. These activities can help clear
your mind and enable you to make a better decision.

10. With some decisions, creating a grid of features
may help. Perhaps you've seen the basic form of a
decision matrix when buying some computer software.

|  | Basic | Deluxe | Premium |
|---|---|---|---|
| Contains Basic Math | X | X | X |
| Contains Alegebra | X | X | X |
| Contains Geometry |  | x | x |
| Contains Calculus |  |  | x |
| Price | $19.95 | $29.95 | $39.95 |

In this first example, if you need calculus instruction, the decision is clear-cut – time to plunk down $39.95 for the premium product. If not, you might want to save some cash and get one of the less expensive programs.

If a more complicated decision is on your plate, such as what job you should take, where you should live or where you should go to college, a more complicated chart may be needed. Let's take the example of a hypothetical student, Jon, who has the choice of attending one of four colleges, each one in a different part of the country. The first step is to list the issues that are important, in this case:

1.  Quality of the physics program

2.  Quality of the literature department

3.  Amount of fun recreation in the town

4.  Quality of the weather

5.  Expense of the college (including living expenses)

6.  Knowing friends that might go to that school

Then set up a graph:

| | Physics | Literature | Recreation | Weather | Expense | Friends |
|---|---|---|---|---|---|---|
| College A | | | | | | |
| College B | | | | | | |
| College C | | | | | | |
| College D | | | | | | |

The next step is to fill in the blanks. In this example, Jon would assign numbers 1 to 5 based on how well each college fares in each category. This is not a 1 to 4 ranking of the four colleges, but, rather, Jon assigned whatever value he thought each the college earned in a given category – for instance, all four colleges could tie in a given attribute. In the case of expenses, the lower price got a higher score.

Before Jon finished, there was another step. All of the categories may not hold the same weight. Although Jon thought it would be nice to have some familiar faces at the new college, the expense of the school and the quality of its physics program was a more important consideration for him. Just as he ranked each college for a given attribute, he then assessed each attribute by giving it a score of 1 to 5.

| | Physics | Literature | Recreation | Weather | Expense | Friends |
|---|---|---|---|---|---|---|
| College A | 5 | 3 | 4 | 2 | 5 | 2 |
| College B | 2 | 5 | 5 | 5 | 2 | 4 |
| College C | 4 | 5 | 3 | 4 | 3 | 1 |
| College D | 3 | 2 | 2 | 1 | 3 | 5 |
| Importance | 5 | 2 | 3 | 2 | 5 | 2 |

On first glance, it might seem that College B is the winner – after all, it has the most 5s. However, when you factor in the importance of each attribute, College A looks pretty impressive. For the fun of it, let's multiply each score by its importance and add them up. I'm not saying this would give Jon an undisputed champ and that he should declare the ultimate winner based on this, but it may be enlightening.

| | Physics | Literature | Recreation | Weather | Expense | Friends | TOTAL |
|---|---|---|---|---|---|---|---|
| College A | 25 | 6 | 12 | 4 | 25 | 4 | 76 |
| College B | 10 | 10 | 15 | 10 | 10 | 8 | 63 |
| College C | 20 | 10 | 9 | 8 | 15 | 2 | 64 |
| College D | 15 | 4 | 6 | 2 | 15 | 10 | 52 |
| Importance | 5 | 2 | 3 | 2 | 5 | 2 | |

Despite College B getting all those 5s, it came in only third place. Jon plans to be a physics major and is on a tight budget, so that improved the ranking for College A.

*Fred had another strategy for dealing with business decisions. Sometimes, two people would offer him a deal and he could accept only one of the offers. He found that letting both parties know when the decision was close often helped him make the decision. One of the parties would frequently go that extra mile for the business deal.*

# 20

# Improve Your Sleep

*"People who say they sleep like a baby usually don't have one."*

Leo J. Burke
Psychologist

I'm not sure why parents feel compelled to offer silly platitudes and pass them off as wisdom, but we do. I guess it's part of the job. So when one of my sons (about 9 years old at the time) was trying to delay his bedtime, I offered up: "You better get to sleep soon, so you can be bright-tailed and bushy-eyed in the morning."

And my son replied, "Dad, I think you're the one who needs some extra sleep." And I probably did.

Relaxation and sleep have an interesting relationship. Adequate sleep is essential for a healthy, relaxed, joyful life. Conversely, you can't fall asleep until you relax. In fact, effort really gets in your way when trying to get to sleep.

Most people at some point or another have come across Chinese finger traps. Put both index fingers in and the more you try to pull your fingers apart, the more the device tightens around your digits. Just relax and bring the tips of your index fingers together and -- voila -- the fingers easily slide out.

When you think of sleep, think of the Chinese finger trap. Getting to sleep by brute force and effort – not very effective. Relaxing and giving into your sleepiness will be much more effective.

Perhaps, you wonder, "Should we forget all this relax-ation stuff and just take a sleeping pill?" In 1991, one research study compared several insomnia treatments. One group received one of the most popularly prescribed sleeping pills of the time (temazepam; brand name, Restoril). A second group was given recommendations for changing their behavior at bedtime, while a third group received both the behavioral recommendations and the medication, and the final group received only a placebo. The only groups with long-term benefit were the groups that were given the behavioral treatments. In a 2006 study, a newer sleeping pill also came up short; behav-ioral measures were more effective than the medication.

How much sleep do you need? The simple answer is that you need enough sleep to feel rested. For some people, that can mean five hours; for others, 10. An average is around eight hours. Some people sleep a little less as they age.

Let's look at some of these important tips for helping you get a good night's sleep so you can feel refreshed in the morning.

## Sleeping Tips:

1. Make your bedroom dark, quiet, and a comfortable temperature; people tend to sleep a little better in cool temperatures. Also, try to reduce clutter around your bedroom.

2. If possible, use the bedroom only for activities such as sleep, meditation, and sex. Avoid eating, doing work activities, or talking on the phone in bed. It is helpful to have your body associate your bedroom with sleep.

3. Avoid caffeine in the afternoon or evening.
   Caffeine can be found in coffee, chocolate, many
   sodas, and caffeinated teas. Certain medications,
   like decongestants, can cause insomnia in some
   people. (Speak with your doctor about other options
   for treating nasal congestion, if needed.) Alcohol
   sometimes helps with getting to sleep initially, but
   it may interfere with the quality of sleep and make
   it more likely that you will awaken in the middle
   of the night.

4. Avoid heavy meals right before bedtime.

5. Regular exercise is important and can help with
   sleep. However, it is best to avoid exercise in the
   two hours just before bed.

6. Establish a bedtime routine, such as taking a bath,
   meditating, or doing another relaxing activity.
   However, after your regular bedtime routine, it is
   often best not to lie down in bed until you actually
   feel a little drowsy.

7. If you tend to worry a lot, write your concerns on
   paper. Such a list can lessen your tendency to think
   about your problems again and again at night.

8. Perhaps most important, don't try too hard. If you
   try to go to sleep for 30 minutes and are still wide
   awake, get up and do something else. You might
   read a boring book with a glass of warm skim milk
   until you feel tired. Then go back to bed. Of course,
   one of the keys is picking a boring book, not a suspense novel. Alternatively, you might try reading
   a magazine article since it has a natural ending

point. It's probably best to pick out an old-fashioned printed book or a black-and-white ink style e-reader. The light from a computer or lit up tablet screen may make it more difficult to drift off to sleep.

9. Try waking up at the same time each morning and getting ready for bed at the same time every night. This schedule can help your body establish a rhythm.

10. If you are having trouble sleeping, try a relaxation exercise. Use meditation to let go of those catastrophizing (and untrue) thoughts that just make the insomnia worse (such as "I'll die without enough sleep," "I'll be useless tomorrow," or "I'll never get to sleep"). Let go of your attempts to fall asleep and just focus on the current breath. Perhaps you can imagine your body sinking into the bed with each exhalation. At times, I find following one breath at a time to be very useful. At other times, I may feel my abdomen expand with each inhalation and relax a muscle group with each exhalation.

   **Optional Audio Exercise:** guided mediation for insomnia available at www.stressremedy.com

11. If the catastrophizing thoughts continue, you can actively dispute them. For instance, you might say to yourself or write down: "I won't die from lack of sleep tonight. Work might be harder if I don't sleep well, but I'll function."

12. What if you have finally fallen asleep and someone or something wakes you up? Well, I can tell you what

does not work. On occasion, someone has mistakenly
called me at 3 a.m. Perhaps a nurse erroneously
thought I was the doctor on call for a problem. I have
learned that it is a mistake to become increasingly
annoyed by being awakened. Then it is tough to get
back to sleep. What works alot better is to handle the
call (or whatever awakens me), roll over, and follow
my breath. I quickly let go of thoughts about why I
should not have been called, or how I really need a
full night's sleep, or how I will be a mess tomorrow.
In other words, I nip my annoyance in the bud and
get back to the breath. In fact, if I wake at anytime
during the night, instead of an attitude of "Oh, no,
I'll be tired if I don't get back to sleep soon," I assume
the attitude of "Perfect time to meditate." In that
way, instead of becoming more frustrated, I can
enjoy a meditation and likely fall off to sleep.

If, despite these recommendations, you still are having
problems with sleep, you can try a modest sleep restriction
and then progressively increase the sleep duration. Set
an alarm to wake up at the same time each morning.
Even if you are tired, avoid napping during the day. If
you think that your ideal amount of sleep to be refreshed
is eight hours, be ready go to bed seven hours before your
time to get up. The next night, go to sleep seven and a
half hours before that time. And the following night, try
going to bed eight hours before that time.

On occasion, almost everyone has trouble sleeping. However, if your insomnia occurs frequently and does not
improve with the above suggestions, you may want to
discuss it with your doctor. Insomnia is sometimes
caused by medical problems. For instance, an enlarged

prostate may cause a man to wake up frequently to urinate. Awakening with shortness of breath is a definite reason to seek a doctor's advice. Clinical depression and anxiety disorders may also cause insomnia and are described in a later chapter.

With sleep apnea, sleeping people may stop breathing for 10 seconds or more at a time. This apnea awakens them long enough to get a breath. People with sleep apnea may wake up more than 100 times a night without being aware of it. Obviously, this frequent awakening causes them considerable fatigue. They may get morning headaches and dry mouth, and high blood pressure as well. Usually, but not always, people with sleep apnea are overweight and snore loudly. Additionally, untreated sleep apnea increases the risk of heart disease, so it is important for people with this problem to seek medical attention.

Restless leg syndrome is another cause of insomnia. When people with this problem go to bed, they feel a need to move or kick their legs, waking up themselves and sometimes their partners. Several medications are useful in treating restless leg syndrome.

If you make the changes recommended in this chapter, both your insomnia and your stress will likely decrease.

# 21

## How Money
## Can Buy Happiness

There is the common phrase that "money can't buy happiness." And indeed, love, joy, and fulfillment are not typically for sale at Walmart, or Tiffany's, for that matter. Or are they? An effective marketing campaign is designed to convince you that what stands between you and your smile is the lack of an Acme watchamacallit. For only "12 easy payments," happiness is yours!

No surprise when Michael I. Norton, an associate professor of business administration in the marketing unit at Harvard business school, wants to convince you that money can buy happiness. A marketing person saying spending money will buy happiness – yawn, yawn – what's new with that? Well ... I'll tell you.

Michael Norton studied people throughout the world and gave them money. Half were instructed to spend the money on themselves; the others were instructed to buy something for someone else. People that spent money on themselves had no significant change in their happiness. However, people that spent money on others were significantly happier.

This shouldn't be surprising. When it came to prehistoric humans, "survival of the fittest" didn't just mean having the biggest biceps. Imagine a group of cavemen who looked out for each other. They were much more likely to survive than cavemen who looked after only themselves. Thereby, as a species, we evolved to find joy in connection and giving to others.

When you review your life to pick out the most relaxed and joyful times, likely you were hanging out with a loved one – hugging your son, holding hands with your significant other, or petting that cute fuzzy puppy.

Another door to relaxation and happiness is through love and connection. We can access this door in two interrelated ways: acting in a giving manner and cultivating feelings of loving kindness.

## Altruistic Giving

If you give for the sole reason of thanks or recognition, you may be disappointed. Conversely, giving something with the sole intent of making someone else happy will likely make you happy.

The beneficial effect of giving is not just relegated to spending money. Spending time and effort may be even more beneficial. In another study involving 2,700 men, the men who did not do volunteer work were two and a half times more likely to die during the study period than the men who volunteered at least once a week.

Besides satisfying our inborn urge to connect and care, making a positive difference in others' lives can bring a sense of perspective to your own life. When you volunteer to help out at the soup kitchen, not having money to remodel your bathroom doesn't seem as important.

*"I don't know what your destiny will be, but one thing I know: The only ones among you who will be truly happy are those who will have sought and found how to serve."*

Albert Schweitzer, physician, philosopher, and medical missionary

*"This is the true joy in life, the being used for a purpose recognized by yourself as a mighty one; the being thoroughly worn out before you are thrown on the scrap heap; the being a force of nature instead of a feverish selfish little clod of ailments and grievances complaining that the world will not devote itself to making you happy."*

George Bernard Shaw, playwright

## LIFESTYLE TIPS

### GIVING TIME, EFFORT AND/OR MONEY

How can you put giving into your week? Are there particular ways that you can give without expectation of reward? What causes are you passionate about? How can you make a difference? Of course there's limit to what you can and should do – balance is important and you also need to also care for yourself. However, you will find reward in following a passion to make a difference in work or with volunteering with friend and family, or with strangers. Sometimes people are overwhelmed by the vast need in the world and then give up on the idea of doing anything. Take a note from Mother Teresa when she said: "If you can't feed a hundred people, then just feed one."

There is a classic story about three brickmasons working on the same job. When asked about his job, the first said, "I have this boring job of placing one brick after another. It is boring, lowly, and demeaning." A second mason said about his job, "The work is solid, and it allows me to provide for my family." When the third mason was asked about his job, he said, "I'm building a cathedral that will last for hundreds – and maybe even thousands – of years. It will offer both physical shelter and spiritual comfort to unknown multitudes. I do my work carefully, because I am so privileged to be a part of this great project."

Although all three masons have the same job, their experience is certainly different. Which one is most stressed and suffering? Which one likely finds passion in

---

**Relax on the Run**

## Focus on the Difference You Make

Pay attention to the difference you make in your current job, home life and/or volunteering. This can make a marked difference in your experience. Also, whatever work you do, do it with integrity and in a way that contributes to others. You can be bored as you sell flowers at a flower stand, or you can seek to make each person you deal with a little happier. Since flowers are often given as presents, you can acknowledge that you are indirectly bringing beauty to people you might never meet. You can struggle working in construction, or like the third mason, you can take pride in acquiring skills and building useful and well-made structures.

his life and thereby works in a relaxed joyful way?

## Cultivating Loving Kindness

Memory and imagination are essential in functioning in day-to-day life and solving intricate problems. By creatively and effectively using our memory and imagination, we can start to access and cultivate feelings

---

**Relax on the Run**

### REMEMBERING LOVE

Right now think about a time when you were feeling very loving and compassionate. I'm not talking about possessive, jealous, or romantic love. I'm referring to the wonderful feeling a parent might have for a child or a pet owner might have for a pet – the feeling that makes you want to do anything for your loved one. After reading this paragraph, close your eyes; remember and visualize a special moment. Perhaps when your child says out of the blue, "I love you," or your dog nuzzles you at just the right time, or your friend says just the right thing to comfort you and gives you a hug. If you don't want to pick out one moment to remember, just close your eyes and imagine seeing and feeling a loved one giving you a hug, or perhaps imagine holding a newborn. Imagine the scene as vividly as possible, noting what you feel, see, and perhaps even some wonderful fragrance.

After doing this, notice how you feel.

---

In 2004, professor of psychiatry and psychology Richard Davidson studied Buddhist monks who were practiced and proficient in a compassion meditation.

The latest equipment, both functional MRI scans and EEGs, was used to study the monks. Results? The measurements were unlike those ever recorded: The monks were off the scale in the areas of happiness and compassion. By regularly practicing a meditation on compassion, they had dramatically changed the way their brains functioned.

By regularly practicing the meditations below, you will actually change your brain to increase happiness and compassion, and decrease stress. (As you learn these meditations, it's worth pondering what the world might be like if more people became adept at these practices.) We spend a lot of time learning a variety of skills, hoping they will bring happiness. Why not spend time practicing skills that are scientifically shown to actually increase

### Practice

## LOVING-KINDNESS MEDITATION

Sit or lie down in a comfortable position. Close your eyes and visualize an image that brings forth loving-kindness. It could be an image of one who has been loving toward you, or it could be the image of holding a newborn in your arms. Imagine the scene as vividly as possible.

Next, visualize a person toward whom you naturally feel affection toward and silently say to that person words such as, "May you be safe and protected. May you be happy. May you be healthy. May you live with ease." (Living with ease does not mean removing all the challenges in life, but rather living joyfully without the sense of struggling.) Say the words at your own pace, and try to say them with meaning. You can modify the wording so that it is most meaningful to you. After you say each phrase, feel the physical and emotional effects of just having said it. If you would like, you can imagine hugging the person or holding his or her hand. Next, say similar phrases to yourself: "May I be safe and protected. May I be happy. May I be healthy. May I live with ease." If it is difficult to direct these phrases to yourself, you can imagine yourself as a small child and say those phrases to that child. Again, after each phrase, feel the effects of the phrase. Then, say the phrases while visualizing someone you might feel more neutral toward, perhaps someone you don't know well. Then say, the phrases to someone you may have had some negative feelings toward. It is probably best not to pick out initially the person for whom you have the most negative feelings. You might start with a person that you have found mildly irritating. Another option is to visualize that person with you and say words such as, "May we be safe and protected. May we be happy," and so on.

Keep in mind that by wishing someone well, you are not necessarily approving that person's behavior. You are acknowledging that all of us really just want to be happy. Sometimes we have been skillful in our attempt – bringing happiness to ourselves and others. Other times, we have been misguided and unskillful – bringing ourselves and others suffering. By keeping in mind our common wish, to just be happy, and our challenges, we can still offer the above wishes.

Traditionally, in a loving-kindness meditation (also known as a Metta meditation) one then offers the same phrases to a whole community and then to all beings. You might take 20 minutes or so to run through the whole sequence as described above. To make it easier to visualize people, you can keep their pictures by you as you do this meditation.

**Optional Audio Exercise:** loving kindness meditation available at www.stressremedy.com

## MINI METTA

Prior to going into an appointment with someone, you might pay mindful attention to a couple of breaths and visualize a loving scene. Then visualize saying "May you be happy and healthy," or other similar phrase, to the person you are about to meet. The 10 or 20 seconds it takes may help your meeting go more smoothly. This exercise is particularly helpful when there has been a history of irritation or tension with another, but it can also be used in any situation.

**Practice**

## COMPASSION MEDIATION

To cultivate compassion toward someone who is suffering, do a similar meditation but imagine the one you know and say phrases such as, "May you be free from suffering and the cause of suffering." Similar phrases can be said to yourself and to all

your happiness? Let's briefly discuss meditations on loving kindness, compassion, and empathetic joy.

## Empathetic Joy

At times, we are distressed by jealousy. Your co-worker gets the raise that you thought you deserved, and you steam. Someone else grabs the parking place that you had your eyes on, and the snake of jealousy bites. A meditation on empathetic joy can be thought of as antivenom for the snakebite of jealousy.

Young children are quite commonly jealous when another gets something. When my twin sons were young, I said to them, "Mommy and Daddy get to be twice as happy as you boys. Would you like to be twice as happy?" That question got their interest. I continued, "When something good happens to me, I get happy. However, I also get happy when something good happens to you. So I can be happy twice as often. You are already happy when something good happens to you. If you want

**Practice**

## EMPATHETIC JOY

When you have more time, close your eyes and visualize someone for whom you care deeply. Imagine saying to that person: "I am happy for you. May your good fortune and happiness continue. May it grow. May it increase." Then, similar to the loving kindness meditation, you can practice saying those phrases to yourself and to others, and eventually to your community and all people.

**Relax on the Run**

## EMPATHETIC JOY

When something good happens to someone else (particularly if you feel jealousy begin to raise its head) say a phrase such as: "I am happy for you" or "That's wonderful!" Depending on the situation, you may say the phrase to yourself or to another, and say it with as much meaning as you can muster.

to be twice as happy, you can also be happy when something good happens to your brother. You can practice this by saying to him, with meaning, 'I am happy for you.'"

If we look closely at our jealousy, we can see how silly it is. People become jealous of others' fame or fortune. When we get to know someone well, we see that those things do not bring happiness. The skills that nurture happiness are the very skills you have been learning to deal with stress. Through mindfulness, empathy, forgiveness, and cultivating compassion, we become more joyful.

# 22
# Wonder and Awe

*"There are only two ways to live your life.*
*One is as though nothing is a miracle.*
*The other is as though everything*
*is a miracle."*
Albert Einstein

*"I didn't say half the crap*
*people said I did."*
Albert Einstein meme

"Wonderful" and "awesome" – words now overused, their meanings diluted to being synonymous with "good." Yet, originally, their meanings must have been more significant, more special. If something was wonderful, it left one full of wonder. Awesome implied inspiring a sense of awe. In these circumstances, instead of being stressed out, we are extremely content.

Whether staring out at the Grand Canyon or looking at your newborn, you likely know that feeling of wonder and awe, a feeling that is, indeed, extraordinarily special. Special, but need it be rare?

How might we have more experiences filled with wonder and awe? How might our lives be truly more wonderful and awesome?

Answer numero uno is our practice of mindfulness; it is difficult, if not impossible, to be in awe while we are judging and complaining. We've reviewed gratitude and loving kindness – two other practices that can deepen a sense of wonder.

Certain words may help evoke these types of experiences as well. Many use the word spiritual to describe experiences of awe. Of course, one's beliefs of spirituality and religion may color the language he or she uses to describe and help bring forth such experiences.

To make things easy to undestand in this chapter, let's categorize people's spiritual/religious beliefs into four broad categories (in no particular order).

Some people believe in a traditional God who is an all-knowing, all-powerful being. If one of these people wanted to recognize and bring forth a feeling of awe and wonder, he or she may look out into nature and see evidence of "God's miracles."

By definition, atheists do not believe in any form of God. Therefore, instead of referencing God, an atheist may look out on a scene and say words such as wondrous, awe-inspiring, or beautiful, and so on. Or one might use knowledge of science to marvel – when admiring scenery, being aware of the vastness of the ocean or of sky; when observing everyday items, pondering the complexity of their atomic structure.

Some people do not consider themselves atheists but they have trouble believing in a God who micromanages the world and determines which baseball team wins the World Series or who gets a job promotion. They have trouble reconciling an all-powerful loving God with the suffering that has been present throughout the history of the world. Yet, because of their spiritual experiences, they may believe in another type of God, one that is so large that He/She encompasses everything – not a manager of events who is separate and above our world, but rather the essence of everything in the world. As opposed to a contrivance, they feel this concept jives with their spiritual experiences, moments when they've felt a special sense of oneness with the universe. These folks may look out into a scene and say to themselves, "God," for to them, there is nothing that is not God. To them, God is everything and recognizing that helps open themselves, to the wonder of the moment.

And there are agnostics, lucky dogs, because they get to chose whichever phrase they like to help describe and promote a sense of wonder. Actually, all of us, whether in the four categories above or in a category I didn't mention, can find the language that works the best for each of us. Although the actual experience of wonder and awe is beyond words, we can all find some words to remind us of what we have experienced in the past, and thusly, remind us of what we can experience right now.

---

**Relax on the Run**

## WONDER AND AWE

Find words or phrases that, for you, best characterize moments of wonder and awe. Occasionally throughout the day, try saying those words to yourself and see if it reminds you to experience the wonder of everyday life.

# 23

# Change

*"When one door closes, another opens;
but often we look so long
at the closed door that we do not see
the one which has opened for us."*
Helen Keller

It is comforting to remember that life's difficulties often eventually work out, one way or another. We have all been upset over a particular event and then later realized that it was actually good fortune in disguise. Not infrequently, I have heard of someone's being laid off from a job only to eventually find a job that was much better.

Some people believe that when circumstances do not look good on the surface, we must trust that there is a larger plan. Having this view helps people cope with disappointment and also decreases worry by increasing confidence that they can handle whatever the future brings. Some people may put this trust in God, and others may trust their own ability to deal with whatever "comes down the pike." Either way, this type of trust can be comforting in times of potential stress.

*Sally told me that, as a young mother, she was overwhelmed with stress. Her young son had been diagnosed with diabetes. This diagnosis required extra care and contributed to extra worry in her already busy life. She was having trouble functioning day to day. Finally, she said, she "gave the problem to God." What I think she meant by that was that she decided to trust that God would help to take care of the situation in one way or another. The solution would all be part of God's plan. Sally worked just as hard providing care to her son, but it was done with less stress. When Sally started to feel too stressed, she would tell herself that she was "giving her problem to God," and she would feel a tremendous sense of relief.*

**"I asked God for strength, that I might achieve;**
**"I was made weak,**
**that I might learn humbly to obey.**
**I asked for health, that I might do greater things;**
**I was given infirmity,**
**that I might do better things.**
**I asked for riches, that I might be happy;**
**I was given poverty, that I might be wise.**
**I asked for power,**
**that I might have the praise of men;**
**I was given weakness,**
**that I might feel the need of God.**
**I asked for all things, that I might enjoy life;**
**I was given life, that I might enjoy all things.**
**I received nothing that I asked for,**
**but everything I had hoped for.**
**Almost despite myself,**
**my unspoken prayers were answered.**
**I am, among all people, most richly blessed."**

Anonymous

You don't have to believe in God to realize that our disappointments may at times bring opportunities.

**"What the caterpillar calls**
**the end of the world,**
**the master calls a butterfly."**

Richard Bach, author

---

**Practice**

# WHEN YOU DIDN'T GET WHAT YOU WANTED

List times that it was good you didn't get what you wanted. A job that you hoped for, but later found out was not for you? A relationship that looked like the best in the universe, but you later found out it didn't look like the thing you so wished for? A loss of a job that ended up leading you to a greater opportunity? List just a few of the best ones:

1. _____

2. _____

3. _____

---

More likely than not, there are many more times you are better off that one of your wishes did not come true. So when life looks disappointing, know that you may not know the whole story.

*My father-in-law was moving from Northern California to Southern California. He rented a truck and a trailer. Just as he was ready to leave, he found that the trailer was incompatible with the truck. As a result, the brake lights wouldn't work. He was forced to leave the trailer in Northern California, knowing that he would need to drive an extra 12 hours round-trip to retrieve it. You can imagine that he might be thinking, "What a catastrophe!" As he set out without the trailer, the truck had a*

*tire blowout. He pulled to the side of the road eas-*
*ily. He later learned that if he had had a blowout*
*while driving with the trailer, his truck would like-*
*ly have jackknifed, and he could have been in a*
*very serious accident. The seeming "catastrophe" of*
*an incompatible trailer might have saved his life.*

Sometimes, a children's story has an important message for adults. In *It Could Have Been Worse*, a young mouse becomes upset on several occasions, as he trips or falls down. He has one mishap after another, so he thinks he is having a terrible day. However, he never seems to notice that each time he falls, it helps him narrowly miss being caught by one of several predators. Each time, he is slightly bruised, but still alive. This story shows children (and their parents) that what seems like an unfortunate event on the surface may, in reality, be a truly fortunate one. Sometimes we, like the mouse, are not aware of the whole story.

And other times, it is hard to think that there could be any silver lining to a particularly nasty dark cloud. And then one takes solace in the fact that things change. Time does not stand still. Life constantly changes. There is an old story of a king who offered an award for a gift that would alleviate his depression when things looked tough and keep him level headed when things looked particularly rosy. A young man won the award by giving the king a box. In the box was a sheet of paper with the phrase, "This, too, shall pass."

## The Final Change

In the midst of a long meditation, sometimes I've pretended that there are only a few moments of the meditation left. In that way, I savor every breath. As I get older, I am more cognizant of how short our lives are. This realization is important, for it encourages us to treasure every moment.

> *"It's only when we truly know and understand that we have a limited time on Earth – and that we have no way of knowing when our time is up – that we will begin to live each day to the fullest, as if it was the only one we had."*

Elisabeth Kubler-Ross, psychiatrist

---

**Relax on the Run**

### YOUR LAST MOMENTS ON EARTH

Whatever you do next, pretend you have only a few moments to live. When you pretend there is time only for this last activity, what is your next hug like? What is that bite of food like? What is the shower like? What is the kiss like? What is that conversation like? Don't just read this, try it now. Notice the level of mindfulness you have. Don't pretend it is your last day; pretend these are your last moments. See how you treasure them. See how you can luxuriate in the moment – how you savor just this step, just this breath.

---

## *Our Ship*

Early this morning,
I cared for a patient with severe dementia.
He, not able to talk or get up out of bed.
And I, not able to ignore or deny
some day, I may be like him.
His hair, salt.
Mine, with some pepper left.
His skin, with furrows;
mine, with lines.
Physical and mental health,
are treated like a given,
but the only real given:
they do not last.
In the past I have actively ignored this,
So not to be depressed by this.
But now it is my bond,
My connection to this person,
And to all people.
We are all on the same ship,
crew-mates on this voyage,
through calm seas,
and rough waters.
The only way the trip makes sense,
is to take it together,
kindly,
connected,
with heart,
courage,
empathy
and love.

by Jay Winner

# 24

# When It's More Than Stress

*"He that won't be counseled can't be helped."*

Benjamin Franklin

The dimly lit Georgetown bar was filled with young men and women, the smell of cigarette smoke, and a cacophony of competing voices. Surrounded by a throng of bodies, my chest became tight and an anxious compulsion grew, driving me down to the first floor of the tavern and then outside to the relatively uncrowded sidewalk. Breathing the cool fresh air, my anxiety quickly dissipated. "What was that?" I wondered. "My first sign of claustrophobia?" My question was not answered for another decade.

Fast forward 10 years: It's New Year's morning and breakfast is served, including a traditional dish of black-eyed peas, allegedly endowing the eater with a year of good luck. In the dining room, we were surrounded by a variety of animals, including dogs, cats, and a lone parrot. Without warning, the very same feeling emerged – the anxious chest tightness, which this time drove me to bid an early farewell to my breakfast companions. At this point, however, I was a young physician and my diagnostic thought process, honed by years of training, guided my next step. I went to my office and placed a tube called a peak flow monitor to my mouth, and forcefully exhaled. Despite using all my effort, the monitor consistently

measure my lung function as barely 2/3 of normal. No –
the problem was not claustrophobia; I had asthma.

Usually, when we feel anxious and stressed we are just
anxious and stressed. However, once in a while, the
stress is just the tip of the iceberg, a symptom of a larger medical issue. Chest tightness could certainly be from
plain vanilla stress, but it would be unwise to count on
that until you checked it out. Chest tightness could also
represent heart disease, anemia, or lung disease – in my
case it was asthma.

The problems in this chapter are not the most common
causes of anxiety but for the most part, neither are they
rare. For instance, if one had a racing heart, weight loss,
anxiety, and a feeling of excessive warmth, it should
make a doctor entertain a particular medical problem.
If that person looked jittery and his eyes bulged as if he
were perpetually surprised – there would be little doubt.
Even a couple of the above features should prompt one
to test for ... hyperthyroidism, a condition in which the
levels of hormone from the thyroid gland is too high.

Anxiety and hyperthyroidism aren't the only conditions
that can make your heart race. If palpitations (racing or
prominent heartbeat) are the most prevalent symptom of
your anxiety, taking your pulse rate during the palpitations and discussing it with your doctor will help clarify
the nature of the problem. See Figure 6 for instructions
on taking your pulse. In general, a resting pulse rate
between 50 and 100 that is regular in rhythm is not
worrisome. An occasional early or late beat – no biggie.
However, if your pulse is irregular or stays above 120 to
130 at rest, medical attention is indicated. A pulse rate
that is consistently between 100 and 120 at rest may

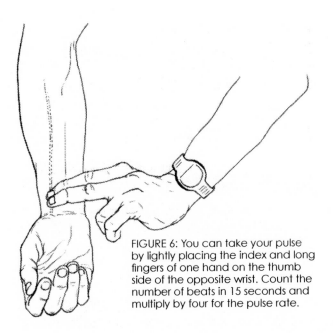

FIGURE 6: You can take your pulse by lightly placing the index and long fingers of one hand on the thumb side of the opposite wrist. Count the number of beats in 15 seconds and multiply by four for the pulse rate.

be the result of anxiety, panic attacks, hyperthyroidism, or just being out of shape. Of course, if you have chest pain or shortness of breath, seek medical attention immediately.

Alcoholism and drug abuse are also associated with excessive amounts of anxiety. In addition, as we covered earlier, caffeine and certain prescription and nonprescription medications can cause anxiety. Common offenders are decongestants, diet pills, and asthma medications. If you are on medication for diabetes, anxiety can result from your blood sugars falling too low. Do not discontinue prescription medications without consulting your health care provider. Abrupt discontinuation of certain medications may also cause temporary anxiety and other more serious problems.

A few other extremely rare medical problems, such as noncancerous adrenal tumors, can cause anxiety. Testing for these problems is necessary only in specific circumstances. (Such circumstances might include anxiety that is associated with very high blood pressure, a racing heart, headache, and feeling flushed.)

## The Anxiety Disorders

Far more common than hyperthyroidism, anxiety disorders affect about 15 percent of the U.S. population. We all have stress, but when the anxiety is so severe or pervasive that it significantly interferes with work or other aspects of your life, you may have an anxiety disorder. To understand anxiety disorders, one needs at least a rudimentary understanding of brain biochemistry.

There are billions of nerve cells in the brain. Messages are transmitted down the length of an individual nerve cell by very small electrical impulses. Between two nerve cells there is a very small space called a synapse. In order for one nerve cell to communicate with another nerve cell, chemical signals called neurotransmitters are released into the synapse.

Altered levels of these neurotransmitters contribute to anxiety disorders or clinical depression. A variety of medications can help with these disorders by regulating the levels of neurotransmitters. Many of these medications are not addictive. Potentially addictive medications may also be beneficial, when used carefully and with appropriate medical supervision.

When they have been diagnosed with other medical problems such as diabetes or heart disease, people usually accept prescribed medication. However, historically, some people have been more reluctant to take medication for anxiety disorders or depression. Does everyone with an anxiety disorder need medication? Of course not.

The situation is similar to type 2 diabetics: Many people with type 2 diabetes can modify their lifestyle – by eating well, getting regular exercise, and losing weight – and by doing so, adequately treat their diabetes without medication. Others can have a perfect diet, run a marathon a day, and weigh less than a  feather, and yet their diabetes is still out of control. If the biochemical abnormality is too great, the healthy choice for the latter folks is to take diabetes medication.

Similarly, many people with anxiety disorders can modify their lifestyle and thought processes – as outlined throughout this book – and by doing so, effectively treat the disorder without medication. Others, although trying their best, may still be incapacitated with fear and anxiety. As with diabetes, if the biochemical abnormality is too great, and the non-pharmacological treatment is not working well enough, medication can make a big difference. Often, the medication is needed only temporarily, giving people the time to build their stress reduction skills; other times the medication is needed long term.

When people have anxiety disorders or depression, it not only affects them; it affects their family, co-workers and friends. (Depression here refers to clinical depression described later in the chapter, not the occasional feelings of sadness that we all have.)

*"The burden of mental illness on health and productivity in the United States and throughout the world has long been underestimated. Data developed by the massive Global Burden of Disease study, conducted by the World Health Organization, the World Bank, and Harvard University, reveal that mental illness, including suicide, accounts for over 15 percent of the burden of disease in established market economies, such as the United States. This is more than the disease burden caused by all cancers."*

National Institute of Mental Health

Although some people worry about long-term negative effects from taking medication for depression and anxiety, there may be long-term effects from not taking medication. Research has shown that depressed people actually have shrinkage in an area of the brain called the hippocampus. Antidepressant medication seems to prevent that shrinkage. I don't want you to become anxious whether you should take anxiety medication. Rather, realize that for each type of mental health disorder there are a variety of effective treatments, some of which employ counseling, and others that also employ medication. A good health care provider can help guide you in your choice.

I'll now briefly review different types of mental health disorders, but enough so that you might be able to recognize a potential problem in you or a friend.

Imagine you're driving along the freeway. Suddenly your heart starts racing, you feel as if you can't breathe, you are shaking, your chest feels uncomfortable, you feel numbness and tingling, and you have thoughts of death. Sound like fun? Hardly, but this may be a typical panic attack for people with panic disorder. Other symptoms may include dizziness, abdominal discomfort, nausea, sweating, choking, flushing, feelings of entrapment, and fears of going crazy or out of control. These attacks often happen for no apparent reason. Sometimes the attacks are so frightening that people develop a fear of going out of the house (a condition called agoraphobia), because they worry that they might have an attack while out. Panic attacks are very treatable with counseling and/or medication. Often a combination of both is most appropriate.

Phobias are exaggerated fears of a specific object or situation. Examples are claustrophobia (fear of closed spaces), fear of high places, and fear of flying. These problems are often alleviated with a short bit of counseling. If someone is scared of flying, they might practice a relaxation exercise while imagining being on a plane, or while in an airport, and actually on a plane. However, if you have an extreme fear of flying and take only one plane trip per year, it may be helpful to take an anti-anxiety medication at the beginning of the flight.

People with obsessive-compulsive disorder, or OCD, are bothered and even disabled by their obsessions and compulsions. Obsessions are recurrent or persistent thoughts that become intrusive. People with these disorders are so disturbed by these thoughts or ideas that they may feel compelled to do certain actions. For instance, they may have recurrent thoughts of being contaminated, compelling them to wash their hands excessively (perhaps even hundreds of times per day). Other obsessions may involve feelings of aggression or of losing control. We have all double-checked that a door is locked or that the stove is turned off. However, in OCD, this checking behavior is excessive and can interfere with functioning. This condition may also be improved with medication and behavioral counseling.

The term generalized anxiety disorder or GAD, refers to excessive anxiety throughout the day as opposed to the intermittent nature of the aniety observed in panic disorder. Social phobia is a persistent fear of certain social situations, such as an immobilizing fear of talking in front of others or of eating in front of others.

Post-traumatic stress disorder (PTSD) became well-known after the Vietnam War. This disorder occurs following a traumatic event that is outside the range of normal human experience. Examples of such traumatic events are war experiences and other violent episodes, such as being raped or witnessing a murder. Some of the more common symptoms of PTSD include having recurring or intrusive recollections of the event, having recurrent disturbing dreams, and being easily startled.

In addition to anxiety disorders, a common medical problem is clinical depression. This is different from occasionally being down or "depressed." In clinical depression, the depressed mood occurs very frequently, for at least two weeks. Activities that formerly brought enjoyment cease to do so or are abandoned entirely. A clinical depression often brings a change in appetite, weight loss or gain, fatigue, and decreased concentration. Other common symptoms are insomnia (especially early-morning awakening with trouble getting back to sleep), trouble concentrating, feelings of worthlessness, excessive guilt, and recurrent thoughts of death.

If you have recurrent thoughts of suicide or if anyone you know starts talking about suicide, immediately seek professional attention. If the situation is emergent, resources include suicide hotlines, calling 911, or going to a local emergency room. If someone starts saying good-byes or starts giving away prized possessions, it can be a red flag. Clinical depression may include feelings of hopelessness and thoughts of never improving. Although depressed people often feel as if their condition will never improve, the vast majority do improve, given time and the appropriate treatments. In these cases, suicide is a truly a permanent solution to a temporary problem.

Why are some people more likely than others to develop depression? Both environmental and genetic factors contribute to anxiety disorders and depression. One study found that people who had a variation in one par-ticular gene were more likely to develop depression when experiencing a given stressful life event.

Seasonal affective disorder, or SAD, is a depression prom-inent in the winter months. This disorder may respond to specifically designed lights.

Given the dramatic hormone and social changes that occur following childbirth, women often experience some sadness or anxiety after having a baby. If this sadness is prolonged and severe, it may be postpartum depres-sion, a temporary condition that usually responds to support groups, counseling, and/or medication. Thyroid disorders are also frequent after a woman gives birth, so in cases of postpartum depression, checking a thyroid blood test often makes sense.

Premenstrual syndrome (PMS), a condition well known to comedians everywhere, is seldom funny if you or your loved one actually has it. Perhaps, because of the comical fame of PMS, doctors now often instead use the term premenstrual dysphoric disorder (PMDD), for this problem that, as both names suggest, describes extreme feelings of depression and anxiety in the days prior to a woman's menstrual cycle. PMS responds to regular exercise and good nutrition, but in more severe cases, medications, such as antidepressants, are very useful.

In bipolar disorder, or manic depressive illness, feelings of depression alternate with "manic" states. Symptoms of mania may include elation, irritability, racing thoughts, and going with little sleep.

If you believe that you or someone you know may have one of these disorders, discuss the issue with a health professional. Appropriate professionals include your family doctor, your internist, or a psychiatrist. Counselors, psychologists, and other qualified therapists may also be helpful, but if medications are needed, you will have to talk with a medical doctor.

*While he was participating in my stress management class, Daniel's stress level significantly improved. Additionally, as he reviewed the class notes, he recognized that for many years he had experienced several of the symptoms associated with clinical depression. He frequently suffered from fatigue, insomnia, decreased sex drive, and a variety of vague physical complaints. He had trouble concentrating and frequently felt sad. He realized that these symptoms had been present to one extent or another for many years. Although the techniques he learned in the class helped, he still felt sad much of the time.*

*For some reason, Daniel had previously seen this sadness as a sign of weakness. Even after learning about the medical syndrome of depression, he was reluctant to seek treatment. Finally, he decided that life was too short not to do what he could to feel better. He went to see his family doctor, who recommended that he start an antidepressant medication and counseling. Daniel was not having much improvement ater six weeks on the antidepressant. His doctor, however, was not discouraged, since he knew that there were 20 antidepressants on the market. Daniel switched to another antidepressant and, after being on the treatment for approximately one month, noticed a dramatic change in how he felt. The fatigue, insomnia, loss of sex drive, sadness, poor concentration, and physical symptoms were all decreased. He finally felt like himself again and he wondered why he had waited so long to seek treatment.*

Do not get me wrong; I am not a "pills-for-everyone" doctor. The vast majority of people do very well without anxiety medication. In fact, as the following story illustrates, many people are prescribed these medicines prematurely.

*Angela was depressed, anxious and didn't want to get out of bed in the mornings. A previous doctor had prescribed an antidepressant. Angela did not like how she felt with the medication, so she stopped it. When Angela visited me, she revealed that she was working her way through college. She spent 15 hours per week in class and needed to study another 15 hours a week. In order to make ends meet financially, she took a job that initially required an additional 20 to 25 hours of work per week. She was doing fine until her boss asked Angela to do a little more work here and there. Before Angela knew it, in addition to her schoolwork, she was working 40 to 50 hours a week at her job – and she was miserable.*

*At our visit, instead of jumping to prescribe another antidepressant, we brainstormed on how she could reduce her work hours. We discussed assertiveness skills and ways she could approach her boss in order to decrease her stress and improve her health. After reducing her work hours, her anxiety markedly improved, and she did well at both work and school.*

We should not rely on medications to cure all our ills. That is one of the very reasons that I wrote this book – to give people a wide variety of non-drug options to deal with stress and anxiety. However, some people do need medications, and for those people, we must remove any stigma associated with them. When medications are used, they should be used in conjunction with, and not instead of, stress management techniques. All medications, including antidepressants and antianxiety medications, have potential risks and side effects. A good health care practitioner can help you weigh the risks and benefits and will closely monitor your progress.

If you have high blood pressure that is not controlled with diet and exercise, take medication before you have a heart attack or stroke. If you have clinical depression or an anxiety disorder and do not get adequate relief with stress management techniques and counseling, seek further help.

# 25

# In Conclusion,
# the Beginning

*"Education is not the filling of a pail,
but the lighting of a fire."*
William Butler Yeats, poet

I like changing things up – I thought about beginning the book with an ending, but the book would've been way too short. However ending the book with a beginning – now there is an idea. Hopefully this book has sparked your curiosity, ignited your interest, and maybe even stoked your passion to learn. In essence, I hope this is truly a beginning of a journey to a happier, more relaxed, and heathier life.

A major part of education is putting the knowledge into practice. Think of two eighth-grade friends, Ted and Phil, who do similarly well in a junior high Spanish class. Ted goes on to other interests leaving Spanish behind, remembering "buenos dias," but not much else. Phil moves to Spain in ninth grade, practicing his new language skills throughout day, every day for the next decade. Even if Phil never took another Spanish class, his daily practice likely rocketed his fluency light-years beyond his old amigo.

If you've read this book, you've now got a good solid base of knowledge about relaxation. Don't let your relaxation skills wither and die like my calculus skills. I did well in

high school calculus, but I don't use calculus at home or
at work, haven't done it in over three decades, and now
don't have the vaguest idea of how to do it. I did only
mediocre in my high school typing class, but I type every day at work and home, have typed regularly over the
past couple of decades, and now type as automatically as
I breathe. Practice makes a difference.

Knowing how to relax is essential for a happy, fulfilled
life. If you want to do well at work and thrive at home,
knowing how to relax is a prerequisite.

It makes sense to learn from people who have mastered
their respective fields. No one is born the greatest ball-
player, musician, scientist, or orator. Thomas Edison
was told by his teachers that he was "too stupid to learn
anything." Michael Jordan was dropped from his high
school basketball team. Just as some of our bodies make it
harder to be an NBA basketball star, some of us may take
more practice to develop and hone our relaxation skills.
But, the key  to being great in any field is "deliberate
practice."

Researchers have shown that the key to effective practice
involves:

1. Repetition
2. Working toward performance that is just above
   your current level of competence. Step by step,
   as you improve, the goal is progressively more
   difficult.
3. Feedback

How can we apply these principles of deliberate practice to relaxation? There is plenty of opportunity for repetition. Most people get stressed off and on throughout

the day. By looking at these times as challenges to apply your stress reduction skills, you will have boatloads of practice. Your first challenge is to practice relaxation skills when things are already going fairly smoothly. Then you might just imagine a stressful event and relax, and so on. Become more proficient in relaxing during progressively more challenging circumstances, and eventually, when the excrement really hits the cooling device, you'll be more prepared.

When things are not going well, life gives you feedback. Something occurred and now you're more frustrated than a bikini salesman in the Antarctic. First step: Relax now. This may mean mindfully feeling your in breath in your abdomen and relaxing muscle groups as you exhale; it might mean assuming the valet pose, or choosing and using the energy you have and going for a run. Step two is give yourself feedback. Next time this situation occurs, how can you improve your response? Are there ways you can reframe a situation in advance or as it happens? Might you list some of your blessings in life, might you set up some reminders to be more mindful? Perhaps you'll skip the evening news, go to bed earlier and wake up earlier so that you don't have to rush as much in the morning. If you know there is a stressful event around the corner, prepare yourself with strategies.

It's not just this chapter that is a beginning. In a very real way, each and every moment is a beginning. Whether you were mindful in the last moment, you can be mindful in this moment – and in staying with the theme of this chapter, explore life with a beginner's mind. Even if you've eaten a thousand raisins, really enjoy this raisin like it was your first. Even if you've walked thousands of miles, enjoy feeling the ground with this step. Even though you've taken innumerable breaths, right now: Notice this one.

If you did or did not feel gratitude in the last hour, you can choose to be grateful now. At any given moment, you can begin reframing, communicating wisely and attaining balance in your life. When you can, slow down, take care of yourself, help others, forgive, and wonder in amazement that you are even alive.

This journey that began with the goal of relaxation is really a journey that brings you to the core of what life is about – an adventure of productivity, joy and love. We do not want to get to our death and find that we never really lived.

The practice you do is not just for yourself. It is for your family, friends, work associates, and community. Each time you respond with less stress and more compassion, the ripples of your actions extend in ways you may never know. A small bit of kindness may change how another feels and acts, and so on and so on, down the line.

With global communication taking place by way of the Internet, over the phone, and in person thanks to air travel, a small act of compassion for your next-door neighbor may positively affect people on the other side of the world. In these times of hostility and violence, peace must begin within our own selves. Only then can these small ripples of compassion extend and create a more peaceful world. Certainly that goal should also stoke your fire to learn, practice, and continue this very important journey.

May you have peace and happiness, and may your friends, family, and all of us have peace and happiness.

## Suggested Reading List

### General Stress Management and Health

*The Wellness Book: The Comprehensive Guide to Maintaining Health and Treating Stress-Related Illness* by Herbert Benson and Eileen M. Stuart.
New York: Simon & Schuster, 1992.

*Don't Sweat the Small Stuff* by Richard Carlson.
New York: Hyperion, 1997.

*Minding the Body, Mending the Mind* by Joan Borysenko. New York: Bantam Books, 1987.

*Managing Stress: Principles for Health and Well-Being,* 8th ed., by Brian Luke Seaward.
Sudbury Mass.: Jones & Bartlett, 2013.

### Mindfulness

*Peace Is Every Step* by Thich Nhat Hanh.
New York: Bantam Books, 1991.

*Full Catastrophe Living* by Jon Kabat-Zinn.
New York: Dell, 1990.

*Wherever You Go. There You Are: Mindfulness Meditation in Everyday Life* by Jon Kabat-Zinn.
New York: Hyperion, 1994.

*Insight Meditation: A Step-By-Step Course on How to Meditate* by Sharon Salzberg and Joseph Goldstein.
Boulder Colo.: Sounds True, 2001.

*Meditation for Beginners* by Jack Kornfield.
Boulder, Colo.: Sounds True, 2004.

*A Mindfulness-Based Stress Reduction Workbook*
by Bob Stahl and Elisha Goldstein.
Oakland, Calif.: New Harbinger Publications, 2010.

## Cognitive Therapy

*Feeling Good* by David Burns.
New York: Avon Books, 1980.

## Type A Personality

*Treating Type A Behavior and Your Heart*
by Meyer Friedman and Diane Ulmer.
New York: Ballantine Books, 1984.

## Lifestyle

*Simplify Your Life* by Elaine St. James.
New York: Hyperion, 1994.

*Margin and The Overload Syndrome* (these books are
available together, in quite small print, or individually)
by Richard Swenson.
Colorado Springs, Colo.: Navpress, 2002.

*Healthy Pleasures* by Robert Ornstein and David Sobel.
New York: Addison-Wesley, 1989.

## Communication

*Messages: The Communication Skills Book*
by Matthew McKay, Martha Davis, and
Patrick Fanning. Oakland, Calif.: New Harbinger, 1995.

*The Basics of Nonviolent Communication*
by Marshall Rosenberg. DVD available at www.cnvc.org.

## Work-Related Stress

*Don't Sweat the Small Stuff at Work*
by Richard Carlson. New York: Hyperion, 1998.

*The Truth about Burnout* by Christina Maslach and
Michael P. Leiter. San Francisco, Calif.: Jossey-Bass,
1997.

## Relationships and Stress

*Don't Sweat the Small Stuff With Your Family*
by Richard Carlson. New York: Hyperion, 1998.

*Love and Survival* by Dean Ornish.
New York: HarperCollins, 1998.

## Anxiety Disorders

*The Anxiety Book* by Jonathan Davidson & Henry Dreher.
New York: Penguin Putnam, 2003.

## Panic Disorder

*Don't Panic* by R. Reid Wilson.
New York: HarperCollins, 1996.

## Depression

*Understanding Depression* by Raymond J. DePaulo and
Leslie Ann Horvitz. Hoboken, N.J.: Wiley, 2002.

*The Mindful Way Through Depression: Freeing Yourself
from Chronic Unhappiness* by J. Mark Williams,
John D. Teasdale, Zindel Segal, and Jon Kabat-Zinn.
New York: Guilford Press, 2007.

*Mindfulness-Based Cognitive Therapy for Depression:*
*a New Approach to Preventing Relapse* by Zindel Segal,
Mark Williams, and John Teasdale.
New York: Guilford Press, 2002.

## Importance of Purpose

*Man's Search for Meaning* by Victor Frankl.
New York: Simon & Schuster, 1959.

## Time Management

*Getting Things Done: The Art of Stress-Free Productivity*
by David Allen. New York: Penguin Books, 2001.

## Raising Children

*Setting Limits with Your Strong-Willed Child:*
*Eliminating Conflict by Establishing Clear, Firm and*
*Respectful Boundaries* by Robert MacKenzie.
New York: Random House, 2001.

*How to Talk So Kids Will Listen and Listen So*
*Kids Will Talk* by Adele Faber and Elaine Mazlish.
New York: Avon Books, 1980.

*Raising Children Compassionately*
by Marshall Rosenberg.
Encinitas, Calif.: PuddleDancer Press, 2005.

## Spirituality and Compassion

*A Path With Heart: A Guide through the Perils and*
*Pitfalls of Spiritual Life* by Jack Kornfield.
New York: Bantam Books, 1993.

## Recommended Websites

Important information on stress, including updates about this book and my related work:
www.stressremedy.com & www.relaxationontherun.com

Finding a counselor specializing in anxiety disorders:
www.treatment.adaa.org/

Information on nonviolent communication:
www.cnvc.org

Meditation retreats: www.spiritrock.org
and www.dharma.org

Mindful eating: www.tcme.org

## Optional Audio Exercises

- Six-Minute Meditation
- One-Minute Relaxation
- Guided Meditation
- Letting-Go Meditation
- Sound, Breath, Body, Thoughts, and Emotions
- Walking Meditation
- Eating Meditation
- Stretching Meditation
- Three-Minute Meditation
- Letting Go and Reframing Exercise
- Loving-Kindness Meditation
- Relaxation Exercise for Insomnia

More information at www.stressremedy.com

# References

## Introduction

*Stress shortening life,* "Caregiving as a Risk Factor for Mortality." Journal of the American Medical Association, Vol. 282, 1999; pp. 2215–2219.

*Stress aging you.* Elissa Epel, Elizabeth, et al., "Accelerated Telomere Shortening in Response to Life Stress," *Proceedings of the National Academy of Sciences,* Vol. 101, No. 49, December 7, 2004, pp. 17312–17315.

*The risk of Alzheimer's disease.* R. S. Wilson, "Proneness to Psychological Distress Is Associated With Risk of Alzheimer's Disease," *Neurology,* Vol. 61, No. 11, December 2003; pp. 1479–1485; and R. S. Wilson, "Proneness to Psychology Distress and Risk of Alzheimer's Disease in a Biracial Community," *Neurology,* Vol. 64, No. 2, pp. 380–382.

## Chapter 2: Good Stress/Bad Stress

*Stress shortening life.* "Caregiving as a Risk Factor for Mortality." *Journal of the American Medical Association,* Vol. 282, 1999; pp. 2215–2219.

*Stress and heart disease.* Mika Kivimaka et al., "Work Stress and Risk of Cardio Vascular Mortality: Prospective Cohort of Industrial Employees," British Medical Journal, Vol. 325, No. 857, October 19, 2002, p. 857Aboa-Éboulé Corine et al., "Job Strain and Risk of Acute Recurrent Coronary Heart Disease Events," *Journal of the American Medical Association,* Vol. 298, No. 14, pp. 1652-1660.

*Stress being the number one impediment to academic success.* ACHNCHA2 Spring 2014 Reference Group Executive Summary. Hanover, MD: American College Health Association. http://www.acha-ncha.org/docs/ACHA-NCHA-II Reference-Group ExecutiveSummary Spring2014.pdf

*How one interprets stress may influence if it is good or bad stress.* J. Jamieson, M. Nock, and W. Mendes. "Mind Over Matter: Reappraising Arousal Improves Cardiovascular and Cognitive Response to Stress." *J Exp Psycholo* Gen. August 2012. 141(3): 417-422.

## Chapter 4: Practice Makes Perfect

*Neuroplasticity.* S. W. Lazar et al., "Meditation Experience Is Associated with Increased Cortical Thickness," *Neuroreport*, Vol. 16, No. 17, November 28, 2005, pp. 1893–1897.

*Calm; smile mantra.* Thich Nhat Hanh, *Present Moment Wonderful Moment.* Berkeley, Calif.: Parallax Press 1990, p. 32.

## Chapter 5: Putting Mindfulness Into Practice

*Putting feelings into words seems to modify the reaction in a part of the brain called the amygdala.* "Feelings Into Words: Affect Labeling Disrupts Amygdala Activity in Response to Affective Stimuli," *Psychological Science*, May 2007, Vol. 18, pp. 421–428.

*As a guide from beyond—RUMI.* Printed with permission of Maypop and Coleman Barks from *Say I Am You: Poetry Interspersed With Stories of Rumi and Shams by Rumi,* translated by John Moyne and Coleman Barks. Athens, Ga.: Maypop, 1994, p. 41.

## Chapter 6: When Mindfulness Seems Difficult

"I'm On Fire" by Bruce Springsteen. Copyright © 1985 Bruce Springsteen (ASCAP). Reprinted by permission. International copyright secured. All rights reserved.

*Three-Minute Breathing Space. Mindfulness-based cognitive therapy, or MBCT.* Zindel Segal, Mark Williams, and John Teasdale, *Mindfulness-Based Cognitive Therapy for Depression: A New Approach to Preventing Relapse.* New York: Guilford Press, 2002. pp.173–175

### Chapter 8: Thoughts on Thoughts

*Nine categories of cognitive distortion.* David D. Burns, *Feeling Good.* New York: Avon Books, 1980, pp. 42–43.

### Chapter 10: More on Thoughts and Imagination

*Visualization you can use to help.* Jack Kornfield, A Path with Heart. New York: Bantam Books, 1993, p. 165.

### Chapter 11: Rushing 'round the Clock

*Story about worn chairs.* Friedman admits to an upholsterer's pointing out the excessive wear but claims that the revelation about the type A personality did not occur until a little later. Meyer Friedman and Diane Ulmer, *Type A Behavior and Your Heart.* New York: Ballantine Books, 1984.

*Risk of developing a heart problem.* I. Kawachi, D. Sparrow, A. Spiro, et al., "A Prospective Study of Anger and Coronary Heart Disease: The Normative Aging Study," *Circulation*, Vol. 94, 1996, pp. 2090–2095.

*Risk of high blood pressure.* Lijing Lan et al., "Psychosocial Factors and Risk of Hypertension and Coronary Artery Risk Development in Young Adults (CARDIA) Study, "*Journal of the American Medical Association*, Vol. 290, 2003, pp. 2138–2148.

*Difficult life of medical residents.* Samuel Shem, The House of God. New York: Dell Books, 1981.

## Chapter 12: Balance and Time

*Social support and resistance to colds.* Sheldon Cohen et al., "Social Ties and Susceptibility to the Common Cold," *Journal of the American Medical Association,* Vol. 277, No. 24, June 25, 1997, pp. 1940–1945.

*Social support and longer life.* J. S. House, K. R. Landis, and D. Umberson, "Social Relationships and Health," *Science,* Vol. 241, 1988, p. 545.

*Incidence of heart disease.* Eugene Braunwald (Ed.), *Heart Disease: A Textbook of Cardiovascular Medicine,* 16th ed. New York: W. B. Saunders, 2001, pp. 2247–2248.

## Chapter 13: Technology

*Television watching, obesity and diabetes.* Frank B. Hu, Tricia Y. Li, Graham A. Colditz, Walter C. Willett, and JoAnn E. Manson, "Television Watching and Other Sedentary Behaviors in Relation to Risk of Obesity and Type 2 Diabetes Mellitus in Women," *Journal of the American Medical Association,* Vol. 289, 2003, pp. 1785–1791.

## Chapter 14: Less Stress Nutrition

*Eat food, not too much, mostly plants.* Michael Pollan, "The Omnivore's Dilemma." New York: Penguin Press, 2006.

*Obesity and insulin resistance.* Damien McNamara, "Regular Breakfast Eaters at Lower Risk for Obesity," *Family Practice News,* May 15, 2003, p. 10.

Kaiser Permanente. *"Keeping a Food Diary Doubles Diet Weight Loss, Study Suggests." Science Daily,* July 8, 2008.

*Over 50 percent of the carbon in their bodies were from corn.* Ian Cheny and Curtis Ellis. *Corn King,* 2007.

## Chapter 15: Less Stress Exercise

*Optimal amount of jogging.* Schnohr, Peter, et.al. "Dose of Jogging and Long-Term Mortality: The Copenhagen City Heart Study," *Journal of the American College of Cardiology,* Vol 65. No. 5, February 10, 2015, pages 411-419.

## Chapter 16: Communication

*One of the most satisfying feelings I know.* Rogers, Carl. *A Way of Being.* Boston: Houghton Mifflin Company, 1980, pp. 22–23.

*Motivation, she felt better.* Adapted from a story by mediator Judith Rubenstein.

## Chapter 17: Communication Part 2

*Take your time.* Rosenberg, Marshall, Ph.D., Raising Children Compassionately. Encinitas, Calif: Puddle Dancer Press, 2005, pp. 9–10.

## Chapter 18: Anger and Frustration

*The country of Tibet was invaded by China* in 1949. Jon Kabat-Zinn, *Wherever You Go There You Are.* New York: Hyperion, 1994, p. 49.

*Once I was traveling to give a lecture.* John-Roger Peter McWilliams, *You Can't Afford the Luxury of a Negative Thought.* Los Angeles: Prelude Press, p. 277.

*Don't ignore the positive.* The Dalai Lama and Howard C. Cutler, *The Art of Happiness.* New York: Riverhead Books, 1998, Chapter 10.

## Chapter 20: Improve Your Sleep

*Behavioral changes vs. pills for insomnia.* C. Morin et al., "Behavioral and Pharmacological Therapies for late-life insomnia: A randomized controlled trial," *Journal of the American Medical Association,* Vol. 281, March 19, 1999, pp. 991–999.

*Behavioral changes vs. pills for insomnia.* B. Siversten et al., "Cognitive Behavioral Therapy vs. Zopiclone for the Treatment of Chronic Primary Insomnia in Older Adults: A Randomized Controlled Trial," *Journal of the American Medical Association,* Vol. 295, June 28, 2006, pp. 2851–2858.

## Chapter 21: How Money Can Buy Happiness

*However, people that spent money on others were significantly happier.* Dunn, Elizabeth W., Lara B. Aknin, and Michael I. Norton. "Prosocial Spending and Happiness: Using Money to Benefit Others Pays Off." *Current Directions in Psychological Science* 23, No. 1 February 2014: 41–47.

*The men who did not do volunteer work were two and a half times more likely to die during the study period than the men who volunteered at least once a week.* Hafen, Brent Q., Keith J. Karrren, Kathryn J. Frandsen, and N. Lee Smith, Mind/Body Health. Boston: Allyn and Bacon, 1996, p.403.

## Chapter 23: Change

*He trips or falls down.* Benjamin, A.H.; Tim Warnes, *It Could Have Been Worse.* Waukesha, WI: Little Tiger Press. 1999.

## Chapter 24: When It's More than Stress

*Antidepressants seemed to prevent shrinkage of hippocampus.* Y. Sheline et al., "Untreated Depression and Hippocampal Volume Loss," *American Journal of Psychiatry,* Vol. 160, 2003, pp.1516–1518.

## Relax on the Run Exercises

**More Relax on the Run
exercises are integrated
into the following chapters:**

## Practice

## Lifestyle Tips

### More Lifestyle Tips are integrated into the following chapters:

Less Stress Nutrition

Less Stress Exercise

Improve Your Sleep

## ACKNOWLEDGEMENTS

I owe a debt of gratitude to the following people: First and foremost, I would like to thank my wonderful wife, Dana, who has provided me with love, support, and advice; and my children, Sam and Zach, who inspire me and continually teach me about life and love.

My parents, Shirley and Seymour Winner, and my sister, Jody Ginsberg, all helped provide a wonderful, loving environment for me to grow up in and continued to offer support and love over the years.

I'd like to offer special thanks to my patients and students, who have taught me so much, and thanks to a variety of authors whose wisdom has been made available to me and others.

I very much appreciate the invaluable inspiration and help provided by my friends. Thank you to my superb co-workers and colleagues at Sansum Clinic. Multiple people, including (but not limited to) Ali Javanbakht, Michelle Robin La, Starshine Roshell, Greg Stathakis, Danielle Kent, and Sierra Huffman, reviewed the material and gave important feedback.

I appreciate the art work of Sam Winner (valet pose) and Susan Meyers (diaphragmatic breathing and taking pulse). Paula Pisani is a talented editor. Her work was stellar, and is much appreciated. Anna Lafferty did a superb job with both the cover and interior book design, and went above and beyond, offering advice on wording as well.

## NOTES

# NOTES